MENOPAUSE WEIGHT LOSS

LIVE WELL, SLEEP WELL, STOP HOT FLASHES & LOSE WEIGHT

JANE THURNELL-READ

CONTENTS

DISCLAIMER

The information in this book is not a substitute for professional advice from your physician or other qualified health care provider. If appropriate, please consult with your own physician or healthcare specialist regarding the suggestions and recommendations made in this book.

Do not disregard professional medical advice or delay in seeking it because of something you have read in this book.

This book is not intended for use by people with eating disorders, unless advised to read it by their health care provider.

Although many people buying this book are native English readers, the way we spell words is not uniform.

I'm based in the UK, so prefer the English spelling. In the UK we talk about hot flushes rather than hot flashes. Yet I've used the North American spelling in the title, because the North American market is so huge compared with other English-speaking countries. So, I've continued to write hot flashes throughout the book itself unless I am quoting research where hot flushes is used. Other than that, I have chosen UK English spelling.

OTHER BOOKS BY THE AUTHOR

All books available on Amazon as paperback and eBooks

"190 Weight Loss Hacks: What the Evidence Says" March 2022
(Also available as an audio book on Amazon, Audible and iTunes)

Specialist Books for CAM Therapists

"Energy Mismatch for Kinesiologists, Dowsers & EAV Practitioners"
November 2021

"Verbal Questioning Skills for Kinesiologists & Dowsers" November
2021

THE EATING OUT ACTION PLAN

Do you struggle when you eat out? Do you end up eating more food than you want? Do you end up feeling weak-willed and fat? Then, is it difficult to get back on track? If this applies to you, my eating out action plan is what you need.

WORRY FREE GUIDE TO EATING OUT

I've brought together a 7-step action plan for when you eat out. Going to a restaurant or a party can be fun, it can also be very stressful, if you want to lose weight or keep off the weight you've already lost.

Each step is carefully explained. There's a bonus cheat sheet to take with you when you go out. You can either download and print it, or just have it accessible on your phone.

Access it here: www.janethurnellread.com/freebie

INFORMATION IN YOUR HANDS
& HOPE IN YOUR HEART

*M*enopause! It can feel like a time when your body and mind are taken over by forces outside of your control. It can feel like everything is changing with no certainty of what the future will hold. It can feel that there is not much you can do about it – you either rail at the sky or accept the situation with as much grace as you can muster.

You may feel that it's all down to your hormones and there's nothing you can do about that. You may think that hormone replacement therapy is the only option. You may feel that your best years are over. It's all downhill from now on.

You may feel angry a lot of the time and defeated some of the time. Maybe you toss and turn in bed, drenched in sweat and gloom.

This book will change how you feel about your menopausal symptoms and your future by putting power and control back in your hands and in your mind.

I will show you that menopause symptoms are a gift to you. They are a message about your life and what you need to do, and to become, to be happy and healthy into old age.

WINDOW OF VULNERABILITY

Researchers call menopause a window of vulnerability when women may be more susceptible to problems.

Barbara Mangweth-Matzek[1] (Innsbruck Medical University, Austria) and colleagues gave an anonymous questionnaire to women aged 40-60. The answers showed that:

"… the menopausal transition is associated with an increased prevalence of eating disorders and negative body image. Menopause, like puberty, may perhaps represent a window of vulnerability to these conditions, likely because of changes in hormonal function, body composition, and conceptions of womanhood."

An article in the academic journal Maturitas[2] says:

"… perimenopause is characterized by estrogen change and may also present a window of vulnerability to eating disorder development."

This is undoubtedly a time when you need to embrace self-care. I hope you are doing that anyway, but often we end up putting everyone else first. Sometimes you have an absolute right to put your own self-care ahead of looking after other people. If you have children, it's good for them to see that you value yourself and your needs. You give them a role model for how they need to look after themselves too.

Understanding that you are in a time of vulnerability as your hormones change gives you the extra impetus you need to take care of yourself at this time.

IS THE UPHEAVAL OF MENOPAUSE BENEFICIAL?

This time of hormonal fluctuations is often seen as a disaster or an insurmountable challenge. But it can be experienced as a beneficial time. It forces many women to prioritise their own self-care. They find they have to put themselves first simply to get through the day. Many women have spent their adult lives being busy, with little time for themselves. Maybe you are one of these women, juggling a career and love for your family (children, spouse, aged parents). This may be the first time you have been forced to really consider your own needs, your own importance. It may be the first time you have really lavished love on yourself.

It's important to see menopause symptoms as messengers reminding you to take care of yourself.

DIFFERENT PLACES, DIFFERENT EXPERIENCES

If you're in the middle of vaginal dryness, brain fog, night sweats and weight gain it can be hard to accept that society and its expectations are playing a part in all this. You can feel like these are completely factual states and that you have no control over them.

Yet research suggests strongly that how women experience menopause is affected by the society they live in.

In an article for the British Psychological Society[3] three psychologists wrote:

"Biologically, something happens to women, but the experience is so diverse that rather than uniting women across the globe, menopause serves to demonstrate how varied the perceptions of physical changes can be. While the majority of women experience menopause as a relatively neutral event, women, living in Western countries tend to report more symptoms."

They point out that Japanese women tend to report headaches, chilliness and shoulder stiffness as the most troublesome menopausal symptoms. Rural Greek women and women in the Mayan culture have been found to report few problems during this time of transition.

In an article in The Conversation[4] Janet Viljoen of Rhodes University (South Africa) points out that studies have found menopause symptoms vary. Aching joints and back pain are more common for white women, whereas African-American women experience more hot flashes and night sweats.

The Physicians Committee for Responsible Medicine[5] (USA) say:

"Hot flashes have been reported by only about 10 percent of women in China, 17.6 percent of women in Singapore and 22.1 percent of women in Japan. In contrast, it is estimated that hot flashes are experienced by 75 percent of women over the age of 50 in the United States."

We do not have certain knowledge of why there are these differences. It's likely that cultural expectations play a part, but it may also be in part down to differences in lifestyle.

It's interesting that women in western countries tend to report more symptoms. Is this because these cultures tend to emphasise more the loss of youth and sexuality? Menopause is "getting old". It can seem altogether less threatening when menopause is seen to mark the transition to a wise and respected elder in the community. The typical western diet is widely regarded by medical experts to be unhealthy. Does this have an effect too?

Even within a society not all women have the same experience of this transition.

A study in the Journal of Women & Aging[6] did in-depth interviews with 48 women. The authors identified three different ways women described menopause:

1. Menopause as a normal, biological process
2. Menopause as struggle, involving identity loss, shame, and a changing place in society
3. Menopause as transformative and liberating

Knowing that some women experience this time as liberating can be depressing and bewildering if debilitating menopause symptoms are ruling your life. It may be that women who experience only minor symptoms experience menopause as transformative and liberating.

You may feel that you can't change the culture you live in, and you can't change the symptoms you are experiencing, so this information is useless! Maybe it's worse than useless, because it makes you feel bad that you aren't sailing through it like those women in the third category.

That is definitely not my intention. I want to open a window where you can see that there is another possibility. Your experience can change. Your perception can change, but not just by wishing it or by will power. You need information that you can use to change how you think about menopausal symptoms and the level of distress you experience.

If you were experiencing very few symptoms, would you feel differently about what is happening to you? The answer is probably yes. So, let's look at how you can change the symptoms and see this as a time of change, some of which will be glorious. Rather than a window of vulnerability could it be a window of opportunity?

 "So many women I've talked to see menopause as an ending. But I've discovered this is your moment to reinvent yourself after years of focusing on the needs of everyone else. It's your opportunity to get clear about what matters to you and then to pursue that with all of your energy, time and talent." Oprah Winfrey

2

WEIGHT GAIN AT MENOPAUSE

or many women weight gain is one of the most distressing menopausal symptoms. It can lead to a loss of confidence. You may feel unattractive, even ugly.

IS WEIGHT GAIN INEVITABLE?

Many women think weight gain is inevitable at this time unless they follow a strict diet and exercise vigorously and obsessively. But is this true? Let's have a look at the evidence.

A study from Monash University[1], Australia compared women who go through an early or late menopause to those who go through menopause normally. They found in all women the weight gain occurred at the same age, showing menopause itself was not the cause.

If menopause hormonal changes caused you to put on weight, you would expect those experiencing early menopause to put on weight much earlier in their lives than those with a late menopause. That didn't happen.

Professor Davis, Director of the Women's Health Group at

Monash, said that the idea menopause causes women to gain weight was A MYTH.

Professor Davis went on to say:

"It is really just a consequence of environmental factors and ageing which cause the weight gain."

A study[2] by Hanna-Kaarina Juppi published in the journal Aging Cell found:

"Higher diet quality and physical activity level were ... inversely associated with several body adiposity measures. Therefore, healthy lifestyle habits before and during menopause might delay the onset of severe metabolic conditions in women."

In other words, eating well and exercising regularly means you are less likely to gain weight or develop diseases such as type 2 diabetes and heart disease.

Researchers from the University of Naples Federico II[3] (Italy) concluded:

"Weight gain is a common phenomenon in menopause and age of onset is influenced by several factors. Among modifiable risk factors are sedentary lifestyle and unhealthy nutritional patterns, which often result in obesity that in turn contributes to an increase in cardiovascular risk in menopause, mostly through low-grade inflammation."

An Australian study[4] based on 7270 women found that around 60% managed to avoid weight gain at menopause. You definitely wouldn't believe the figure is that high from media reports and advertising.

Clare Collins, Professor in Nutrition and Dietetics, University of Newcastle (UK) and colleagues writing in The Conversation[5] agree:

"Even though weight gain is common, you can beat it by using menopause as an opportunity to reset your eating and exercise habits."

This insight from Professor Collins supports what I said

earlier – this is a time to have a big reset, changing your lifestyle to something that will serve you for the rest of your life.

DOES WEIGHT AFFECT MENOPAUSAL SYMPTOMS?

In a study of 929 Korean women, researchers[6] found that obese women had more frequent menopausal symptoms than normal or overweight women. WHO defines overweight as a BMI (body mass index) greater than or equal to 25 and obesity is a BMI greater than or equal to 30. There are lots of body mass index calculators on the internet. Just search "BMI calculator" if you want to know your BMI.

Other studies have agreed with these findings, such as a study of Brazilian women[7]. 749 Brazilian women aged 45 to 60 years showed that obese women suffered more severe consequences of hot flashes. The researchers write:

"... body-fat tissue acts as a strong heat insulator. The insulation makes the distribution of heat more difficult, which then causes obese women to suffer more hot flashes. The associations between an increased BMI and other symptoms, such as joint and muscular pain and more intense urinary problems, were also confirmed."

In the same article Dr JoAnn Pinkerton, executive director of The North American Menopause Society is quoted as saying:

"In some studies, but not all, weight loss and exercise have both been shown to reduce hot flashes in women who are obese, thus giving women even more reason to create a healthier lifestyle for themselves."

So, putting on weight at this time is likely to make some of your menopause symptoms worse.

IS MY WEIGHT GAIN A RESULT OF BLOATING/WATER RETENTION?

Water retention is associated with changes in sex hormone levels. For this reason, some women experience water retention during menopause. It's also associated with an increase in salt in the diet.

Weight gain because of water retention is usually temporary with your weight fluctuating sometimes by as much as several pounds. Real weight gain tends to occur slowly and be less subject to fluctuations. It's important not to lull yourself into a belief that your weight gain is temporary water retention when it clearly isn't.

Bloating can also be caused by eating too quickly or eating things that do not agree with you. It can also be caused by swallowing too much air. This can be a sign of a digestive illness. If it continues, check it out with your health provider. Air swallowing can also be a reaction to psychological stress. If this is likely, look at what you can do to reduce your stress levels.

MENOPAUSE & YOUR SHAPE

I started to talk about this on a webinar and said: "fat moves". One of the participants said: "Yes, my fat jiggles around!" We all fell about laughing, even though everyone knew this wasn't what I meant.

A review of the literature published in the journal Climacteric[8] found that weight gain itself cannot be attributed to the transition, but it does lead to an increase in abdominal fat.

Your belly is more prone to weight gain during menopause. This is because of hormonal changes. There is a higher testosterone-to-oestrogen ratio. This alters where the body deposits fat. Fat comes off the hips and is deposited around the middle.

This can mean you "feel fatter". When you sit down, an extra two pounds on your belly is much more noticeable than the two pounds that have come off your hips.

A study published in the academic journal Menopause[9] looked at 749 women aged 45 to 60 years. They found that: "menopausal symptoms, including vasomotor, joint, and urinary symptoms, were related to obesity. Hot flashes were associated with higher body mass index, urinary urgency, and vaginal dryness."

In other words, weighing less means that you are less likely to suffer from typical menopause symptoms.

AGEING & WEIGHT GAIN

We've seen that research confirms it's not menopausal changes themselves that cause weight gain. It's part of the general ageing process. But why would ageing increase your weight?

As you age, your body starts to work less efficiently. Muscle mass starts to decrease. When that happens, your body burns fewer calories at rest. This means you need fewer calories overall.

If you continue eating and drinking as you've always done, you will gain weight. That is unless you make other lifestyle changes.

If it's any consolation, this also happens to men, because (remember) it's not about the female hormonal changes!

You may be someone who doesn't mind that you've put on a few pounds. You may feel that there are more important and interesting things to focus on than what you weigh. I agree, but carrying a lot of excess weight rather than a few extra pounds has implications for your long-term health.

You may be thinking that even though menopausal changes aren't driving this, the outcome is still the same – obsessive food control and horrendous amounts of unpleasant exercising to keep your weight stable.

But it's really important that you understand what is going on with your body. If you believe it's "all hormonal", then it's easy to attribute weight gain to factors beyond your control. If you believe your hormones are responsible, you don't do anything about it (other than curse your hormones) when you put on two pounds.

If you understand that weight gain at this time is not because of hormonal changes, you will want to look at your diet and lifestyle to see what has changed.

Your weight gain may be because you've started drinking more wine in the evening or having cookies with your morning coffee. Maybe you're watching more television or using the car more. Maybe you think that now you're getting older you need to take it easy. You may feel you can afford (and deserve) those expensive cakes. Whatever age you are, these small changes will lead you to put on weight.

Believing that your weight increase is down to your hormones, and that you can't do anything about it becomes a self-fulfilling prophecy. This quote sums it up:

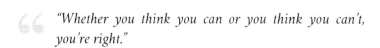

> "Whether you think you can or you think you can't, you're right."

Henry Ford

Don't worry. I'm going to explain later how to lose that pesky weight you're putting on. For now, just understand that it's not all about hormone changes. It's not something that you just have to accept. You have agency. You have power.

3

AM I TOO OLD TO CHANGE?

*O*nly you know the answer to this. It depends on your mindset. If you feel that you're too old to change and it's pointless, you'll struggle to lose weight and have a healthy lifestyle. But the evidence does support the idea that you can lose weight and get healthier – if you want to and believe it's possible.

A study[1] from the University of Warwick and University Hospitals Coventry and Warwickshire (UHCW) NHS Trust demonstrates that age is no barrier to losing weight. The study looked at patients attending a hospital-based obesity service and found there was no difference in weight loss between those under 60 years old, and those from 60 to 78 years old.

Lead author Dr Thomas Barber of Warwick Medical School at the University of Warwick said:

"Weight loss is important at any age, but as we get older we're more likely to develop the weight-related co-morbidities of obesity. Many of these are similar to the effects of aging, so you could argue that the relevance of weight loss becomes heightened as we get older, and this is something that we should embrace."

Research also encourages exercise for healthy later years. Sadly, many people are frightened they might injure themselves if they start exercising later in life. But the evidence suggests exercise can help prevent injury, even if started later in life.

In a study published in Frontiers in Physiology[2], researchers in the University of Birmingham's School of Sport and Exercise Science (UK) compared muscle-building ability in two groups of older men. The first group were classed as 'master athletes' -- people in their 70s and 80s who are lifelong exercisers and still competing at top levels in their sport. In the second were healthy individuals of a similar age, who had never participated in structured exercise programmes. Lead researcher, Dr Leigh Breen, said:

"Our study clearly shows that it doesn't matter if you haven't been a regular exerciser throughout your life, you can still derive benefit from exercise whenever you start ... Obviously a long term commitment to good health and exercise is the best approach to achieve whole-body health, but even starting later on in life will help delay age-related frailty and muscle weakness."

The Victoria State Government website[3] (Australia) encourages older people to exercise but says this:

"If you develop any new symptoms after you start getting active, see your doctor straight away. New symptoms could include:

- Dizziness
- Chest pain
- Shortness of breath
- Unplanned weight loss
- Sores that won't heal
- Pain anywhere in your body

"Discontinue exercising until you've seen your doctor and worked out what is causing your symptoms."

Although exercise is triggering the symptoms, it's showing up an underlying problem.

Bear this in mind, but also accept that if you want to lose weight and get fit, age is no barrier. In fact, I believe that the evidence confirms losing excess weight and being fit are even more important when you're in the second half of your life than they are when you are younger.

You may be reading this and thinking that you've never had a healthy lifestyle, so where to begin? Change can feel challenging, whatever your age. Recognise that it's normal to feel hesitant and uncertain when you start to make lifestyle changes. It's often easier, and in the long run better, to make one or two small changes. As these become part of your life and you begin to feel more confident, add in other changes too.

I absolutely promise you that the rewards you will get from adopting a healthier lifestyle will amaze you. They will have benefits in all aspects of your life – not just for any current weight gain. I also promise you that you will wish you'd started it all a lot earlier in your life.

I know this from personal experience. I hated exercise as a child. I was the only one in my primary class that couldn't touch their toes. In senior school I found everyone could stand on one leg, but I couldn't. The only team sport I remotely enjoyed was hockey, because this allowed me "accidently" to hit another classmate who had annoyed me. In my twenties I was vegetarian, but my diet consisted of toast and marmalade, coffee, orange juice and chocolate. I also drank around a quarter of bottle of whisky a day and regularly smoked at least 40 cigarettes a day. Eventually I started to change and reap the benefits of a better lifestyle.

I believe you can do this too.

4

WOULDN'T IT BE EASIER JUST TO TAKE HRT?

*H*RT is hailed as a wonder drug, and it certainly appears to be that for many women. Some women feel they get back their body, their mind and their life once they start it.

A review of the literature published in the journal Climacteric[1] found that:

"There is strong evidence that estrogen therapy may partly prevent this menopause-related change in body composition and the associated metabolic sequelae."

They are clear in the article that it doesn't necessarily lead to a reduction in overall weight but stops its re-distribution on to the belly.

There have been some concerns raised about the safety of menopausal hormone therapy. It's generally agreed that taking an oestrogen-progesterone combination of HRT gives you a small increased risk of breast cancer.

The most definitive study[2] to look at the safety of hormone therapy is from the Women's Health Initiative study. 27,347 participants were divided into two groups. One group received HRT and the other group a placebo. The study lasted for five to seven years. The researchers followed up the study and found that there was no variation in death rates between the two groups.

The UK NHS website[3] says:

"HRT does not significantly increase the risk of cardiovascular disease (including heart disease and strokes) when started before 60 years of age, and may reduce your risk.

"Taking HRT tablets is associated with a small increase in the risk of stroke, but the risk of stroke for women under age 60 is generally very low, so the overall risk is still small."

Studies[4] looking at whether HRT can reduce women's risk of dementia have been inconclusive.

The research suggests that HRT is effective for some menopausal symptoms and has very few health concerns.

Yet HRT like most drugs is designed to fix a specific problem – common menopausal symptoms such as hot flashes, vaginal discomfort, bone loss, etc. Taking HRT doesn't turn your lifestyle into a healthy one. It doesn't prevent you developing type 2 diabetes, heart problems. It doesn't stop you becoming frail and dependent. It doesn't delay dementia. A healthy lifestyle can do all of this and more.

Rather than seeing menopause symptoms as something to eradicate, see this time as a wake-up call to get your life in order for the rest of your life.

People are living longer, but they are not necessarily experiencing those extra years as healthy years. A European Union survey[5] found that on average people had around 80% of their life as healthy life years.

"In 2019, the number of healthy life years at birth was estimated at 65.1 years for women and 64.2 years for men in the EU, this represented approximately 77.5 % and 81.8 % of the total life expectancy for women and men."

"Wellness is not a 'medical fix' but a way of living - a lifestyle sensitive and responsive to all the dimensions of body, mind, and spirit, an approach to life we each design to achieve our highest potential for well-being now and forever." Robert C Anderson

Taking HRT may well reduce your unpleasant menopause symptoms, but it won't increase the percentage of healthy life years you have. It's not designed to do that.

If you feel you need to take HRT, discuss it with your doctor. If you find that taking HRT reduces or eliminates troubling symptoms don't be lulled into thinking you don't need to look at your lifestyle. You absolutely do, because you need to ensure that you have as many healthy life years as possible.

Of course, some reduction in healthy life years is caused by poverty, genetics and other factors. We can't control everything. But most of us can control a lot of how we experience later life.

So, I want to show you how you can change your lifestyle, without giving up joy. In the process you'll almost certainly experience fewer menopause symptoms. You'll also almost certainly experience better health, wellbeing and happiness as you age. HRT Doesn't promise that!

You may say that you can take HRT and address important lifestyle changes at the same time. If that's realistic, go for it.

You may recognise that you need to make lifestyle changes, but you find your menopause symptoms so debilitating that you don't have the strength to make them. It may make sense for you to take HRT to reduce or eliminate your menopause symptoms, but before you make that decision check out the rest of this book. If you still feel you need to take HRT, at least in the short-run, commit yourself absolutely to revisiting all the information in this book when you've got debilitating symptoms under control.

You need and deserve to be healthy and happy well into old

age. It's not just down to luck. It's something you are almost certainly going to need to work at, but the rewards are immense.

I like this description of what we need to do from Professor Clare Collins[6] (University of Newcastle, UK):

"it's like having to do a spring clean on your life stage patterns, on your dietary patterns and on your physical activity. And you can get through menopause in a healthy weight and with a healthy lifestyle and be healthier. But we have to be on guard."

If you are already taking HRT and now want to stop, please consult your doctor or other qualified health professional first.

5

HOW TO AVOID MENOPAUSE WEIGHT GAIN

*S*o, we've established that hormonal changes of menopause don't cause weight gain. Changes in muscle mass, activity levels, diet etc. do.

We know that weight gain at this time and later in life is not inevitable for the vast majority of women. So, the big question is how to prevent the weight gain.

When I talk to friends who've never had a problem with their weight, they say something like: "Well, it's easy. You just need to eat less and take some exercise." They often believe that people who are over-weight are weak willed and greedy, or else they are stupid. They need to get a grip!

For some people losing weight is straight forward. They decide they want to lose weight, go on a diet, lose the weight and then stabilise at a lower weight. The fact that you've bought this book suggests you are not one of these people! You may be putting on weight now or maybe you've always struggled with your weight.

You may find it offensive that people think it's easy to lose weight. It implies you're being lazy, idiotic or weak-willed if you are overweight.

The good news is that a lot of the strategies you need to lose weight and keep it off are also strategies to live a happier and healthier life. You'll be healthier because you weigh less, but more importantly you'll be feeding your body the right foods to keep you healthy into your old age.

You'll be happier too, not just because you've lost the weight. Many of the strategies you use to lose weight are also strategies you can use to gain more control of other aspects of your life too. For instance, learning to monitor your hunger levels can help you to be more attuned to other changes in your body.

DO I JUST NEED WILL POWER?

Knowing all this can be empowering. It means you can do something about that weight gain. In this book we discuss the changes you need to make, including to your diet and exercise routine. Your heart may drop at the thought of changing your lifestyle so much. If you hate exercise and vegetables, you may feel that you're doomed to put on weight.

But I want to show you that it doesn't have to be some strict and joyless life.

It's also not all about will power. I'm not saying: "It's simple. Just start eating better and exercising more."

Research[1] in the *European Journal of Personality* has shown that people who believe that willpower is limited, tend to exert less self-control through the day than people who believe it isn't limited. Put simply, if you believe willpower is limited, it is!

Later in the day you may be tired. Research suggests when you're tired, you make poor choices. When you're stressed or ill, you make poor lifestyle choices. This isn't about willpower. It's about everything else that is going on in your life. Rather than trying to summon more willpower, see if you can make changes to reduce your tiredness and stress.

IT'S NOT JUST ABOUT WEIGHT

If you're suffering from night sweats and sleeping badly, it's very normal to want to reach for sugary treats to get you through the next day. If you feel that you are losing a vital and important part of yourself as you age, it's not surprising that you comfort eat. If you have children, but they're now independent, you may feel lonely and bored. Maybe food is trying to fill that emotional hole.

Mayo Clinic (USA) researchers reviewed the weight gain risks and challenges faced by women in midlife. Ekta Kapoor[2], a Mayo Clinic endocrinologist and the study's lead author said:

"This population of women faces multiple challenges for maintaining a healthy weight ... Mood changes, sleep disturbances, hot flashes and the many other changes of menopause can disrupt what may have previously been a healthy lifestyle."

Ther main title of this book is Menopause Weight Loss, but this is not a diet book. Focussing on diet alone is like trying to fit yourself into a dress that is too tight. Reducing hot flashes, sleeping better, exercising and finding more reasons to be happy will reduce your desire for comfort food and make losing or keeping weight off that much easier.

Of course, if you haven't had a healthy lifestyle in the past, menopausal changes can make it even more unbalanced. But remember, this book is about hope and solid actionable information. The first step was buying this book. You can change your lifestyle for the better. There are more steps ahead of you. Embrace the challenge and go forward.

6

HOW CAN I AVOID REGAINING WEIGHT?

*Y*ou may be wondering why I'm writing about weight maintenance before explaining how to lose weight. Surely you need to lose weight first, then worry about maintaining the weight you've lost. Isn't it putting the cart before the horse?

If this is the first time you've tried to lose weight, working on weight loss seems the first thing to do. Working out how to maintain the weight you've lost can come later.

But you are probably not in that situation. You may be reading this book and reflecting on how many times you've lost weight only to regain it. Weight loss maintenance is very difficult for many women, regardless of their age. This can make the idea of trying to lose weight again deeply depressing. It's hard to feel enthusiastic and determined if all the struggle in the past has eventually led you to regain all the weight, and maybe even some more.

Traci Mann[1], professor of psychology at the University of Minnesota (USA) analysed every randomised controlled trial of diets that included a follow-up of at least two years. She concluded:

"The dieters had little benefit to show for their efforts, and the non-dieters did not seem harmed by their lack of effort. In sum, it appears that weight regain is the typical long-term response to dieting, rather than the exception."

This is so depressing. And maybe you have come to this conclusion yourself, when you look back at your weight loss attempts. You may now feel that you don't stand any chance of maintaining your weight. I hope to show you that it can be done. It takes work, but it also takes a different approach to what you've tried before.

That's why I've put weight loss maintenance before losing weight. I want you to feel confident that when you get to a weight that works for you, you will have strategies you can use to help you maintain what you have lost. If you don't have this confidence, a little voice will constantly be telling you that there's no point in losing weight, because you'll just put it all back on again.

Of course, there are women who have never worried about their weight, but they are now concerned about how they will maintain their existing weight because of all the dire stories they have heard. If you're in this situation, this section is for you too.

Part of the reason many women struggle to maintain the weight they've lost is that getting to that weight has involved a lot of denial. Losing weight can strongly reinforce the benefit of that denial. The scales and their clothes say this strategy is worthwhile. But now at their working weight, they have nothing further to show for their denial. Staying the same is really not a strong motivator for most of us, whereas losing weight can be exciting and heady stuff. It's not surprising that a large percentage of women put the weight back on.

So part of the strategy to maintain weight is to avoid the denial route to weight loss. Yes, you can lose weight without feeling that you have to deny yourself all the time. I'll explain how later.

There has been a lot of research on long-term weight maintenance. There are several strategies that have been shown to be highly effective.

The first is self-monitoring. I'm a huge fan of this one, as it helps me maintain my weight within a small window without getting stressed out. I weigh myself every day at the same time.

Personally, I don't write it down, but you could if you wanted to. It may be helpful to tell someone else every day what you weigh. It may not be helpful. Experiment to see what works for you.

It's important to understand that you are looking for trends. If I appear to have put a pound on one day, no worries. If it's still there the next day, time to make a mental note. If it's still there on the third day, I start to look at what has changed. It may have been that we've had visitors and my weight will go down again once they've left. I don't need to do anything, except keep a close eye on what happens to my weight once they've left. If there isn't anything special happening, I will think about what I am eating and whether I have been allowing extra unhealthy food to creep in. If that's the case, what do I need to do about it? Have I been drinking more alcohol? Why is that? How can I go back to what it was before when my weight was stable?

My weight tends to be naturally fairly stable. When I was younger, it would fluctuate much more. I could "put on" four pounds (two kilo) from one day to the next. If you are like this, you wouldn't start to question whether you were gaining weight, until more days have passed.

With this approach I'm not thinking about being "good" or "bad" depending on what the scales say. I'm monitoring my weight and problem-solving if it starts to creep up. And I'm solving small problems, so I don't need to go on a rigid diet or deprive myself and come up with big solutions. I just need to make small changes every now and then to stay on course.

I prefer weighing daily to weekly, which some authorities recommend. If I weighed myself weekly, it would be several weeks before I could be certain that my weight gain wasn't a normal fluctuation but was an actual gain.

As well as weight loss, you need to think about exercise. Do I hear you groan? There is a whole chapter of this book on exercise, including how to learn to enjoy it if you hate it.

Research from the University of Colorado[2] (USA) found:

"… successful weight-loss maintainers rely on physical activity to remain in energy balance (rather than chronic restriction of dietary intake) to avoid weight regain. In the study, successful weight-loss maintainers are individuals who maintain a reduced body weight of 30 pounds or more for over a year."

Another important strategy is having an eating plan that works for you. One that allows you to enjoy food, fills you up and gives you energy, good health and a sense of well-being. It's also one that has room for some foods and drinks that have no nutritional value, but that you enjoy. Guess what? This is the diet plan you need to be following to lose that excess weight in the first place.

7

CHANGING YOUR DIET

J've been talking about changing your diet, but what exactly do I mean? The first thing to notice is that I'm saying, "change your diet" not "go on a diet". These are very different things.

Sadly, we have all been encouraged to believe that if we want to lose weight, we need to go on a diet. But that's not what I'm advocating. Going on a diet means that one day (possibly quite soon) you'll come off the diet.

It's important that as you lose weight, your new diet becomes embedded in your life. If you follow any diet where you lose weight, you will experience some immediate benefits, such as less skin chafing and clothes fitting more comfortably. If you follow the best dietary strategy to lose weight, you will also find many other benefits. These come from feeding your body the right nutrition. The benefits include fewer headaches, better sleep, a more optimistic mood, and just more zest for life. There are also long-term benefits, which we are often unaware of. In following a highly nutritious diet we reduce the likelihood that we will develop type 2 diabetes and other chronic health problems.

If you want to improve your diet, change slowly. Focus On Nutrition (Harvard Medical School) says:

"By the time you are 40, you'll have eaten some 40,000 meals —and lots of snacks besides. Give yourself time to change, targeting one item a week… Take a long-range view. Don't get down on yourself if you slip up or "cheat" from time to time. Don't worry about every meal, much less every mouthful. Your nutritional peaks and valleys will balance out if your overall dietary pattern is sound."

The first strategies involve eating and drinking more. I've deliberately put these first as it's important to start with increasing rather than restricting. It's a way of getting away from that diet mentality that may have had you in its damaging grip. It's easy to believe that to lose weight, you have to give up things. I want to start by looking at adding things.

Don't tackle all the diet changes at once. Give yourself time to make one normal before you move on to the next. That way you won't get overwhelmed, and you will make progress.

DRINK MORE

Water is really important to the body. It can also help you eat less, particularly if you drink water before meals. Elizabeth A Dennis[1] and colleagues conducted an experiment in which half the participants drank 500 ml (1.06 US pints) of water before meals. After 12 weeks weight loss was around 2 kg (4.4 lbs) greater in the water group than in the non-water group. This was a 44% greater reduction in weight over the 12 weeks for participants who drank water before meals. All the participants were middle-aged and older adults and followed a low-calorie diet for the 12 weeks.

This is a significant amount of additional weight loss for something that is cheap and easy to apply. I definitely suggest this is the first thing you change about your diet.

It's also worth having a glass of water at other times. If you are feeling peckish, try having some water, wait a while and then see if you are still hungry.

EAT MORE

I'm not telling you to eat more doughnuts or more calories generally. The first focus, particularly if you've been dieting a lot in the past, is to eat more vegetables.

Most people don't eat enough vegetables. Eating more veggies has also been shown to be an effective part of a strategy to deal with menopausal symptoms.

A study of 400 postmenopausal women[2] in Iran divided the women into three groups according to their normal diet:

1. Eating a lot of vegetables and fruit (VF)
2. Eating mayonnaise, liquid oils, sweets, and desserts (MLSD)
3. Eating solid fats and snacks (SFS)

The researchers found that those women following a diet with a lot of fruit and vegetables had fewer menopausal symptoms than the other two groups. Vegetables can fill you without adding lots of calories. Fruit can make excellent snacks.

In another study[3] comparing perimenopausal women who were vegans and omnivores, the researchers found that vegans reported fewer bothersome physical symptoms, including hot flashes and night sweats:

"... more vegetables and less flesh food were associated with less bothersome symptoms."

When we think of vegetables, we often think of fresh vegetables, but frozen or canned count too. Vegetable smoothies can also play a role, if you like them.

A diet high in vegetables can be really beneficial for weight control. It can also help prevent or delay dementia, a common fear as women get older. UK polls[4] suggest that dementia has become the most feared health condition among people over the age of 50, even more than they fear heart disease, cancer and stroke. But guess what? Eating a diet rich in veggies can also lower your risk of heart disease and some cancers.

While, right now, you may be focused on taking action to reduce those pesky menopausal symptoms, know that you are also taking action to increase the likelihood of having a healthy old age too.

ADD FIBRE

Fibre doesn't contain any nutrition and at one time was dismissed by nutritionists as having nothing of value in it. But over recent years fibre has been seen to be vitally important to your health and well-being.

Foods that are high in fibre include wholemeal bread, brown rice, fruit, vegetables and legumes/beans. To add more fibre to your diet, move to wholegrain carbs (at least some of the time). Add beans and peas to your meals. You can have baked beans on toast or add beans to a chilli or a curry. Eat whole fruit rather than relying on fruit juice.

Fibre in the diet can help you to feel fuller for longer, meaning that it's easier to control what you eat. It also means that your blood sugar is less likely to spike. When blood sugar spikes, you are likely to get mood swings. You may feel irritable, shaky or angry. These are not good emotions when you are trying to lose weight.

Carbohydrates have got a bad name – they are seen to be fattening. This is of course true for carbohydrates such as sugar.

But some carbohydrates contain lots of great fibre and include a range of vitamins and minerals as well.

It's also important to consider the food's glycaemic index. Each food containing carbohydrates has been given a score to show how quickly that food affects your blood sugar (glucose) level when that food is eaten on its own. Low glycaemic index foods cause your blood sugar levels to rise and fall slowly. This may help you feel fuller for longer. Low glycaemic index foods include wholegrain foods, fruit, vegetables, beans and lentils. High glycaemic foods include sugar and sugary foods, sugary soft drinks, white bread, potatoes and white rice.

An Iranian study[5] of 393 postmenopausal women concluded that women who ate higher-quality carbohydrate [low glycaemic index and containing lots of fibre] had fewer physical and psychological symptoms of menopause. Similar results were found in a study in Ghana[6].

In another study Kim, Yunsun MD and colleagues analysed the data[7] from 5,807 women collected via the Korea National Health and Nutritional Examination Survey in 2014, 2016, and 2018. Fibre intake was assessed by asking the women what they had eaten in the previous 24 hours. The women also completed a patient health questionnaire. The researchers found that premenopausal women were less likely to be depressed if they ate adequate amounts of fibre. It made no difference for the postmenopausal women.

If you're premenopausal, you will definitely want to be sure to have an adequate fibre intake. Even if you're postmenopausal, you will still want to ensure you have enough fibre in your diet. Adequate fibre reduces constipation, helps you to feel fuller on fewer calories and is protective against some cancers.

What's adequate fibre? If you eat a lot of vegetables, beans, whole fruit and wholemeal grains (breakfast cereal, bread, pasta, rice), you won't have to worry about getting adequate levels of fibre in your diet.

ADD IN SOME NUTS AND SEEDS

If you have been calorie counting, you may be horrified at the idea of adding nuts, because they are such a high calorie food. Yet researchers[8] analysed US data from three longitudinal studies of health professionals. Their results were published in the *BMJ Nutrition, Prevention & Health*. They concluded that:

"... increasing daily consumption of nuts is associated with less long-term weight gain and a lower risk of obesity in adults. Replacing 0.5 servings/day of less healthful foods with nuts [14 g/0.5 oz] may be a simple strategy to help prevent gradual long-term weight gain and obesity."

Other studies have shown the same thing. Eating nuts and seeds, preferably whole rather than processed, is beneficial for health and does not lead to weight gain.

INCREASE FOOD DENSITY

Food density is another way of thinking about what you eat. The result is the same. You will eat more fruit, legumes and vegetables if you follow my recommendation not to be dense!

But what does that mean? Food density, also called calorie density, is a measure of the number of calories in a given weight of food. Doughnuts have a higher density than apples. If you ate the same weight of apples and doughnuts, you'd be eating a lot more calories from the doughnuts than you would be from eating the apple. That's calorie density.

By frequently choosing low density foods you will be eating a lot more food by weight but not by calories. This helps you feel full while losing weight. Low density foods also tend to have a higher nutrient content. They have vitamins, minerals and other substances that help us look good and feel good. High density foods can make us spotty and bad tempered.

The US Centers For Disease Control (CDC) in a booklet called "More Volume, Fewer Calories" offers this advice:

- Add water to your meals via soups and stews
- Drink smaller portions of fruit juice by adding water
- Add fruit to your meal to increase water and fibre
- Begin your meal with a salad.
- Add legumes (beans/pulses) to your meals
- Use whole grains
- Use nuts in small quantities

The Mediterranean diet places an emphasis on the consumption of vegetables, fruits, whole grains, legumes, herbs and virgin olive oil. It doesn't eliminate meat or dairy, but it's much lower than in the typical western diet.

Six researchers wrote in Europe PMC[9]:

"It has been observed that greater adherence to the MedD [Mediterranean Diet] in menopause is associated with reduced risk for becoming overweight/obese, better cardiometabolic profile, and an improvement in menopausal symptoms."

LOOK AFTER YOUR BUGS

The gut biome consists of all the bacteria that live in our gut. They digest the food that we lack enzymes for. The gut biome is, of course, important for your digestion. It's also been shown to be important for your immune system. Some research is now suggesting that your gut bacteria can affect what you weigh and how easily you lose weight. We can't be certain of this, because it's difficult to determine which comes first – being overweight or having particular gut bacteria.

Oluf Pedersen, professor of Metabolic Genetics at the Novo Nordisk Foundation Center for Basic Metabolic Research at the University of Copenhagen[10] (Denmark) and his team analysed the gut bacteria of 123 non-obese and 169 obese adults, and found that the 23% of those who had a comparatively low diversity were more likely to be obese, have insulin resistance and elevated blood lipids, and increased levels of inflammation markers in the blood, all of which increase the risk of type 2 diabetes and cardiovascular disease. Those who were both obese and had lower bacterial diversity gained much more weight over the previous nine years.

Guess what? If you want diverse gut bacteria (and you do), you can achieve that by eating more vegetables, legumes, whole grains (brown rice, wholemeal bread, etc.) Is this sounding familiar?

Tim Spector[11], professor of genetic epidemiology at King's College London (UK) says:

"... if you want richer microbes, you'll eat more of a range of foods and that will induce chemicals that will calm you."

If you were calmer, would you do less stress eating? Almost certainly. So, this is yet another reason to eat to give yourself a variety of gut bacteria.

Researchers at the American Gut Project found that people who ate more than 30 different plant foods each week had a more diverse gut microbiome compared with those who ate 10 or fewer. The World Cancer Research Fund website[12] has an excellent summary of what this means. They divide fruits and vegetables into these groups:

- Fruit and vegetables, each fruit and vegetables count as one food. So, if you have lettuce twice in a week, it's still only counts as one of your 30 different plants
- Legumes, such as beans, such as black, cannellini or kidney, chickpeas, and lentils.

- Grains: oats, buckwheat, millet, wheat, brown rice, wholemeal pasta and quinoa. White pasta and rice aren't included, because the industrial processes used to remove the wholegrains strip them of many of their nutritional benefits.
- Nuts and seeds, such as almonds, hazelnuts, sunflower seeds, pumpkin seeds.
- Herbs and spices: they're plant-based but, because the quantities we eat tend to be fairly small, each is only counted as one-quarter.

This information is on an important cancer research website, because this is an important part of cancer prevention – eating a varied diet that includes a lot of plants. But it doesn't stop there. Eating like this will support your gut biome, which affects your immune system. You may be focussed on making changes because you want to lose weight, but rest assured at the same time you'll be helping yourself in all sorts of other ways.

Are you beginning to feel that all roads are leading to Rome? Whether I'm talking about food density or fibre or eating more, or the Mediterranean diet or the gut biome the conclusion is the same – eat more vegetables and more whole grains.

SUGAR & FAT

Sadly, for many years, researchers who were supported by the sugar industry told dieters they needed to focus on reducing fat in their diet. They were told that fat is the real culprit. Manufacturers responded by reducing fat in their products, but to maintain the taste increased sugar and salt instead.

We now know that fat is not the enemy. Many fats are needed for good health. The Harvard Health Blog[13] says:

"… don't be afraid to go back to fat. Just make sure it's the healthy fats like avocado, olive oil, and nuts. Don't cut out the fat, and don't make a habit of eating products labeled "fat free.""

Melina Jampolis[14], M.D., is a board-certified physician nutrition specialist, specialising in nutrition for weight loss and disease prevention. She says:

"You need healthy fat to absorb the fat-soluble nutrients in fruits and vegetables. You need it for satiety. So I don't tell people to cut fat. But never eat fat alone. Always combine it with a lower calorie density food. If you think like that and get in the habit of doing that, you will be more mindlessly able to manage your weight and optimize your health."

The problem with sugar is that it tastes good and is harmful in all but small quantities. In 1972 John Yudkin, professor of nutrition, wrote a book called "Pure, White and Deadly". That just about sums it up.

Eating sugar can result in a spike in your blood sugar and then later a drop below normal level. Some research[15] has suggested that hot flashes are linked to drops in blood sugar. Avoiding or limiting the amount of sugar you eat may help reduce the number of hot flashes you experience.

Some people find it better to avoid sugar altogether. Others are able to eat some occasionally. You may need to wean yourself off it, gradually reducing the amount you have. As with all the other dietary changes, reducing or eliminating sugar will not only help you to lose weight, it will also reduce your susceptibility to other problems such as diabetes, heart disease and tooth decay.

"Eating crappy food isn't a reward - it's a punishment."
Drew Carey

95 PERCENT DIET

I follow a 95% diet. By that I mean I follow a diet that 95% of the time consists of healthy food. The other 5% can be whatever I want. I find this helps me eat well most of the time, but avoids putting pressure on myself when I don't eat well. I don't actually do the calculations, but it's a useful guide in my mind about how my diet should be. Thinking about what I eat in this way means I no longer stuff myself because I've eaten a bar of chocolate or because I've broken my diet in some other way. Now I enjoy unhealthy food some of the time. I just don't make a habit of it.

EAT MORE VARIETY

You may have read all that I've written and thought that's great, but how do I actually do that? How do I resist all those wonderful delights that the world offers me? As the 95% diet suggests, you don't need to do it all the time, but you do need to do it most of the time. But resisting temptation is hard, sometimes it's impossible in spite of all your good intentions. There is a simple way that will really help you.

It's called the variety effect. If you have a large variety of a particular food, you are likely to eat more. So, you are likely to eat more of a box of doughnuts if they have different toppings than if they all have the same topping. If you feel you need to have unhealthy food in the house for other people, reduce the variety on offer. They will probably unconsciously eat less, and you are likely to be less tempted. But do ask yourself if you are doing them any favours buying this sort of stuff.

I hope by now you are wanting to eat more fruit and veggies, but you may be finding it difficult. The variety effect can help you out here. If you have more variety, you are likely to eat more. Try increasing the variety of healthy food (fruit, vegetables, beans, nuts and seeds) that you have in your house. Have several different types of fruit. Don't just buy one type of tinned beans, have a variety. The more variety you have within a category of food, the more you are likely to eat of that category.

It's a really simple but effective strategy. Buy more variety of the food that you want to eat more of. Buy less variety of the categories of food you are trying to reduce,

SOYA & PLANT OESTROGENS

Plant oestrogens are also called phytoestrogens. Although they are found naturally in plants, they are similar to human oestrogen. They can have an oestrogen-like effect, which could be helpful as women's oestrogen levels decline.

The Association of UK Dietitians[16] (BDA) says that "for some women these effects could be sufficient to help relieve menopausal symptoms, particularly hot flushes." They go on to say that it can take two or three months to see the benefit, and that it's best to eat the plant oestrogens several times a day rather than just once a day.

The BDA also says that consuming more plant oestrogens doesn't help all women, but once again many foods that are high in plant oestrogens are good for us for other reasons. Even if eating them doesn't help your menopausal symptoms, do continue because they will benefit your health in other ways, particularly your heart health.

A study, published by the North American Menopause Society in the journal Menopause[17], found a plant-based diet rich in soy reduces moderate-to-severe hot flashes by 84%, from nearly five per day to fewer than one per day. During the 12-week study, nearly 60% of women became totally free of moderate-to-severe hot flashes. Overall hot flashes (including mild ones) decreased by 79%. The researchers concluded:

"The combination of a low-fat, vegan diet and whole

soybeans (half a cup or 86 g) was associated with reduced frequency and severity of hot flashes and improved quality of life in vasomotor, psychosocial, physical, and sexual domains in postmenopausal women. During the 12-week study period, the majority of intervention-group participants became free of moderate-to-severe hot flashes."

If this result was attributable to a drug, it would be hailed as a wonder drug.

The best sources of plant oestrogens are soya products and flax seed, also known as linseed. Soya products include soya beans (also known as edamame beans), tofu, tempeh, soya milk and soya mince.

Flax seeds have a tough outer husk. If eaten whole, they are likely to pass straight through you, so you won't get any benefit. Most people eat it milled, so the husks are broken down. This allows the body to access the nutrients inside the seeds. Easy ways to take flax seed include adding a tablespoon of it to your morning cereal, adding some when you bake, sprinkling into yoghurt or mixing with mayonnaise for a salad or sandwich. It has a slightly nutty, bitter flavour. In large quantities this would be unpleasant, but in smaller quantities it's fine.

The value of flax seed is not just restricted to hot flashes. A study[18] of Native American postmenopausal women found that regular consumption of flax seed reduced their risk of cardio-vascular disease as seen from lowered LDL-C ("bad choles-terol") and total cholesterol levels.

Flax seed is also thought to be protective against breast cancer[19], so this is another reason to add flax seed to your diet. Flax seed is high in fibre, adding extra benefits to taking it. Make sure you have some fluids around the same time, as the flax seed will need water to swell up.

The National Center for Complementary & Integrative Health[20] (USA) is less convinced about the value of soy products for menopausal symptoms:

"A 2016 systematic review and meta-analysis of 62 studies involving 6,653 women found that specific phytoestrogen supplementations, such as soy isoflavones, were associated with modest reductions in the frequency of hot flashes and vaginal dryness but no significant reduction in night sweats. However, many of the studies included in the review were of low quality.

"A 2018 systematic review and meta-analysis found that soy showed no significant effect on sexual function in menopausal women."

There has been some research that suggests soya might be harmful. The World Cancer Research Fund[21] reviews the evidence and concludes:

"Population studies don't consistently link eating soy with increased risk of any cancer … For now, there is no reason to steer clear of soy, and there is also no reason to consider it a must-have if you prefer not to include it in your diet."

CAFFEINE

A study[22] analysed questionnaires from 1,806 women, who had expressed concern about menopausal problems. The analysis showed that there was a statistically significant link between high caffeine consumption and greater vasomotor disturbance in postmenopausal women. Vasomotor disturbances are hot flashes and night sweats.

Another study[23] found that there was a link between a high consumption of caffeinated beverages and hot flashes.

So how much caffeine is there in various drinks? The amount of caffeine varies between drinks quite considerably, and these figures for different types of beverages and chocolate can only be a guide. Tea that has been brewed longer will contain more caffeine than a cup of weak tea.

The Mayo Clinic[24] has some quite detailed information on this, based on a cup serving of 8 oz or 237 ml:

- regular brewed coffee 96 mg of caffeine
- decaffeinated brewed coffee 2 mg of caffeine
- instant coffee 62 mg of caffeine
- instant decaf coffee 2 mg of caffeine
- black tea 47 mg of caffeine
- cola 22 mg of caffeine
- energy drink 71.9 mg of caffeine

But when you look at figures for coffee chains, it's much more. Larger sizes are often 300 to 400 mg of caffeine.

Check out caffeineinformer.com[25] to find how much is in your favourite brew. The site also includes information on the caffeine content of soft drinks and energy drinks. The USDA[26] calculates that there is 12.4 mg of caffeine in 1 tablespoon (5.4 gr) of cocoa powder. The exact amount of caffeine in a chocolate bar will depend on how much raw chocolate there is in it. White chocolate doesn't have any.

So, should you reduce or eliminate your consumption of caffeine? Reducing a heavy intake of caffeine may reduce the number of hot flashes and night sweats that you suffer from. Even if it doesn't, there are other reasons to consider reducing your caffeine intake.

Caffeine also binds with some minerals (particularly iron) and so stops their absorption. If you are short of iron, avoid caffeinated drinks with meals. Do not take a supplement containing iron with a cup of tea or coffee.

Researchers from the University of South Australia[27] used data from over 300,000 participants in the UK Biobank. They found that too much coffee can increase the risk of osteoarthritis, arthropathy (joint disease) and obesity. In earlier research conducted by the same team six cups of coffee a day were considered the upper limit of safe consumption. They don't say what type of coffee this is or the size of the cup!

In another study[28] the researchers found that high coffee

consumption is associated with smaller total brain volumes and an increased risk of dementia. The researchers set a limit at six cups a day. Obviously if you drink your coffee very strong or in large cups, this figure is less.

All this suggests you should keep an eye on your consumption of caffeine. It may increase the number of hot flashes and night sweats you experience if you start drinking more. Excessive coffee intake is also implicated in dementia, which many postmenopausal women are anxious about.

So what is an excessive amounts of coffee? Dr Astrid Nehlig[29], research director of the French medical research institute, Inserm, and one of the world's leading researchers into coffee, health and brain function says:

"Research shows adults shouldn't go over 400mg a day, which is 4-5 small cups, and no more than 200mg in one sitting."

This really puts into perspective the very large coffees served by the big coffee chains. Think about changing to decaffeinated coffee for some of your consumption. When making coffee at home, replace some of your normal coffee with a high-quality decaffeinated version in your brew.

ALCOHOL

Many women start to drink more around this time, because of the stress and depression they experience related to various symptoms. Some women will also drink more in an attempt to improve their sleep. Stress and depression related to menopause may trigger the onset of alcohol abuse or worsen established alcohol misuse.

Research shows that while alcohol may help you get to sleep, it disturbs the quality of your sleep, so may contribute to your feeling tired the next day.

Alcohol Change UK[30] says:

"Depression is one of the most common mental health problems, with around one in ten people suffering in the UK in any year. Depression and heavy drinking have a mutually reinforcing relationship – meaning that either condition increases a person's chances of experiencing the other."

.The UK Mental Health Foundation[31] recognises the effect on mental health. The website says:

"We often drink alcohol to change our mood. Some people drink to deal with fear or loneliness, but the effect is only temporary.

"When the drink wears off, you feel worse because of the way alcohol withdrawal symptoms affect your brain and the rest of your body. Drinking is not a good way to manage difficult feelings.

"Apart from the damage too much alcohol can do to your body, you would need more and more alcohol each time to feel the same short-term boost. There are healthier ways of coping with tough times."

"For that reason, managing your alcohol intake is one way of reducing your risk of developing depression. If you do experience depression, reducing the amount you drink may help to manage symptoms."

It's not just its effect on depression. Alcohol can have a damaging effect on other aspects of your health.

A study[32] from the World Health Organization's (WHO) International Agency for Research on Cancer (IARC), published in the journal *Lancet Oncology*, has found an association between alcohol and a substantially higher risk of several forms of cancer, including breast, colon, and oral cancers. Increased risk was evident *even among light to moderate drinkers* (up to two drinks a day), who represented 1 in 7 of all new cancers in 2020 and more than 100,000 cases worldwide.

John Hopkins Medicine[33] says:

Heavy drinking ... is linked to a number of poor health

outcomes, including heart conditions. Excessive alcohol intake can lead to high blood pressure, heart failure or stroke."

The North American Menopause Society[34] says:

"Drinking may trigger hot flashes for some women, although that isn't based in research. So determine whether it's a personal trigger for you."

A study by Chrissy Schilling[35] of the University of Maryland School of Medicine (USA) and colleagues concluded:

"The results of this study suggest that light, infrequent alcohol consumption may benefit some women experiencing hot flashes. Future studies should be conducted to confirm our findings and focus on the mechanism by which alcohol use could affect the risk of hot flashes."

Do remember that this research is talking about the benefits of light and infrequent use. Don't use this as an excuse to drink alcohol regularly.

SALT

Many highly processed foods have a high salt intake. Add to that some salted nuts and salted chips/crisps and it's easy to have a high salt intake, even if you don't add much to food. Does it matter?

A study[36] of 9526 women in Korea looked at salt intake for pre- and postmenopausal women. The researchers found that high sodium intake was negatively associated with bone mineral content and bone mineral density in postmenopausal women. This would make postmenopausal women with a high salt intake susceptible to osteoporosis.

The number of women who have high blood pressure increases after menopause. It's believed that female hormones have a protective effect. Research suggests that after menopause blood pressure is affected more by a high salt intake. The mechanism for this is not fully understood.

Here's another quote that you might want to write out and put somewhere prominent:

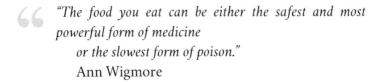

"The food you eat can be either the safest and most powerful form of medicine
or the slowest form of poison."
Ann Wigmore

8

BEHAVIOURAL CHANGE & MINDSET

I have written a book called "190 Weight Loss Hacks: What The Evidence Says" that goes into this in lots of detail. It has been really well received by experts such as doctors and nutritionists.

I don't want to repeat all these ideas and insights here, but I do want to pick out some to get you started. It's unlikely that they will all work for you but do give each one a go and see what happens. Changing your diet can be as much about changing related behaviour or even finding small strategies to move your relationship with food forward.

INCREASE YOUR SELF CONTROL

A study in the *Journal of Consumer Research*[1] says firming your muscles can increase your self-control. I love this idea, because it's so easy to apply. When you are tempted to eat that extra cookie or buy a calorie-busting coffee concoction, just squeeze a muscle. You can make a fist or squeeze your toes or any other muscles – whatever works for you. What about tensing muscles while you look at a restaurant menu? A simple strategy that's been shown to be effective.

MAKE A CONTRACT WITH YOURSELF

The US Centers For Disease Control[2] suggests that you may find it helpful to make a contract with yourself. Write what you intend to do and the behaviour you will consistently maintain, and sign the contract.

FIND YOUR SELF-RESPECT

 "Eating well is a form of self-respect."

I don't know who said this originally, but it's a succinct quote that gets to the heart of things. You could say this every morning before you get out of bed. You could try saying it last thing at night before you go to sleep. What about saying it before meals? You could write it on sticky notes and put them in strategic places. You could turn it into a screen saver. The possibilities are endless. See what you can do with this great quote.

HALT

Halt is a useful acronym to help reduce your eating. It's used by many people recovering from addictions. Here's what HALT stands for:

- Hungry
- Angry
- Lonely
- Tired

When you are reaching for a snack or more food off the restaurant buffet, say "HALT" to yourself. Ask yourself why you are about to eat. Is it because you are hungry? Is it because you are angry? Is it because you are lonely or tired? You only need to go on to eat if you are hungry. Otherwise, you can stop and no harm will come to you! If you are eating because you are angry, lonely, or tired, different strategies are needed.

There are other reasons for eating when you are not hungry – habit is a common one as is boredom. If these sometimes apply to you say HALT and then ask yourself the six possibilities

- Hungry
- Angry
- Lonely
- Tired
- Habit
- Boredom

Once again – only hunger means eat. If the answer is one of the other possibilities, you need to think of other things you can do. In the moment that may be difficult. Eating occasionally because you're angry or lonely or out of habit may well not be a problem. If you find you habitually eat because you're lonely, for example, you need to find other strategies that you can turn to, or maybe you need to think about what changes you need to make in your life.

Here's another great quote:

> "Don't allow a love problem or work problem to become an eating problem. Stop trying to stuff your feelings down with food." – Karen Salmansohn

MINDFULNESS

Mindfulness has become popular as a way of self-calming and gaining more control of your life. The practice focuses on deliberately bringing your attention into the present moment without judgement. Many people find a mindfulness approach helps to change their thoughts and behaviours around food.

It's important to understand that it's not about forcing yourself to behave in a certain way or setting restrictions on what you do. It's about learning to understand and recognise your relationship with food at any time without judging or criticising yourself.

You approach how you think and how you act with compassion and curiosity. You are aiming to stay fully in the present, so that you are not mindlessly eating while you watch a film or talk to friends. Mindfulness can give you the space in which to decide that you're not hungry. It creates a space in which you can change your behaviour, rather than mindlessly pushing food into your mouth.

There is a lot of information about mindfulness on the web. There are also specific apps that help you practice mindfulness on a daily basis. I particularly like the Headspace app[3]. This has a series specifically on mindful eating and another on coping with cravings, as well as more general ones on anxiety, relationship break ups, etc.

In my book "190 Weight Loss Hacks: What The Evidence Says[4]" I discuss how effective mindfulness is in helping people to lose weight. The results seem in general to support mindfulness as part of an overall strategy. On its own it can encourage moderate weight loss, but, possibly more important, it can reduce negative behaviour such as binge eating and food obsessions.

If you want to get a taste of mindfulness, try the raisin exercise. Professor Jon Kabat-Zinn offers a detailed script for this – you can find it on his website mbsrtraining.com[5]. He has it as an audio track and as a written script. The script starts:

"Place a few raisins in your hand. If you don't have raisins, any food will do. Imagine that you have just come to Earth from a distant planet without such food. Now, with this food in hand, you can begin to explore it with all of your senses."

This short exercise encourages you to be present with what you are eating. It shows you how you can learn to eat more mindfully – not just raisins but everything else. You may be surprised at just how satisfied you feel after eating a raisin in this way.

A similar system to mindfulness is Intuitive Eating. This system was created in 1995 by two registered dietitians, Evelyn Tribole and Elyse Resch, based on their extensive experience working with clients. You can find more about it on their website www.intuitiveeating.org[6].

SLOW YOUR EATING

Practicing mindfulness can help slow your eating, which can be really beneficial. A study by Dr Alexander Kokkinos[7] and colleagues of Laiko General Hospital in Athens (Greece) provides a possible explanation for the relationship between speed eating and overeating. Their research showed that the rate at which someone eats may impact the release of gut hormones that signal the brain to stop eating.

Eating slowly can be surprisingly difficult if you've always eaten quickly. My brother says he eats quickly because I used to steal his food as a child!

Maybe you need some help. Try one or more of these:

- Play calming music while you eat

- Put a post-it note on the table reminding yourself to eat slowly.
- Remove bills etc. from the table.
- Put your phone or tablet away.
- Put your cutlery down between mouthfuls, rather than using the time while you're eating to load up your fork or spoon with the next mouthful.
- Eat with a friend who eats slowly.

HABITS

As people get older, they often eat more and more out of habit – they know what they like and what suits them. They may eat according to the clock. When asked; "Are you hungry?", they may immediately look at a watch or clock to decide the answer. Because it's 11 am, do you decide that you'll have a milky coffee and a couple of cookies? That's just what happens at 11am. Do you always have a pudding or other dessert with your dinner? Do you always have bread with soup? Do you always have a bar of chocolate or a couple of glasses of wine of an evening?

Perhaps we shouldn't call it a decision, as it's so automatic. When someone asks you if you are hungry, don't look at your watch, but check out how you feel. What is your digestive system telling you? When you notice it's your normal lunch time, stop and think what you want to eat according to how hungry you are. This will take practice and perseverance.

So, try committing yourself to cooking one new healthy meal a week. If you mainly buy your meals ready cooked, commit to choosing something new each week. If you regularly eat out, try something different from the menu at least once a month. Not everything will be a success, but this way you keep your culinary horizons expanded, and that helps to keep your mental horizons expanded too. These actions will start to break up those automatic eating habits.

Here's a great quote about habits:

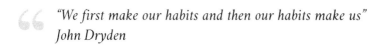

> *"We first make our habits and then our habits make us"*
> *John Dryden*

9

EXERCISE

*M*any women see exercise as solely a means to control their weight. And research[1] has shown that women who maintain or increase their level of physical activity during menopause tend to come out the other end without gaining weight. However, I totally agree with Michelle Segar[2]. She has written the highly popular book "No Sweat." She says:

"If I've said it once, I've said it a thousand times: Exercising for the primary goal of losing weight will not help most people stick with exercise over time. It may get you to start, but it most likely sets you up to exercise in ways that you don't like. As a result, you'll stop once you get tired of forcing yourself to adhere to this regimen and feel like a failure – again. Not only do you not achieve your weight-loss goal, but you also miss out on the multitude of benefits of being active."

There are many other benefits. Here are some startling statistics from the UK National Health Service (NHS) about the benefits of exercise:

"It's medically proven that people who do regular physical activity have:

- up to a 35% lower risk of coronary heart disease and stroke
- up to a 50% lower risk of type 2 diabetes
- up to a 50% lower risk of colon cancer
- up to a 20% lower risk of breast cancer
- a 30% lower risk of early death
- up to an 83% lower risk of osteoarthritis
- up to a 68% lower risk of hip fracture
- a 30% lower risk of falls (among older adults)
- up to a 30% lower risk of depression
- up to a 30% lower risk of dementia"

These are extraordinary statistics. They come from the NHS, an organisation not known for making outlandish, unsubstantiated claims! Sadly, very recently this information has been removed from their website. I don't know why this is. It may be that they felt that the percentage figures were more precise than the research warranted.

But what about exercise and menopausal symptoms? If you are experiencing hot flashes, you may well feel that exercise is the last thing you want to do. Exercise makes you sweaty and hot. But some research shows that exercise is beneficial for hot flash reduction.

Steriani Elavsky, assistant professor of kinesiology at Penn State University[3] USA Says:

"In general, women who are relatively inactive or are overweight or obese tend to have a risk of increased symptoms of perceived hot flashes."

Elavsky and colleagues studied 92 menopausal women for 15 days. They found that (on average) the women in the study experienced fewer hot flash symptoms after exercising. However, the women who were classified as overweight, having a lower level of fitness or were experiencing more frequent or more intense hot flashes, noticed the smallest reduction in symptoms.

Yet there is other research that has shown that exercise can make hot flashes worse or that it has no effect, so what should you do?

Doctors Barbara Sternfeld and Sheila Dugan believe in the importance of exercise. In the academic journal Obstetrics And Gynecology Clinics Of North America[4] they extensively review the literature and write:

"Even if regular physical activity does not prevent or treat VMS [hot flashes and night sweats], the other health benefits that it confers on midlife women will ensure both a healthy menopausal transition and healthy aging."

In the same article they say:

"Another significant benefit of regular physical activity is enhanced mental health, including protection against the onset of depressive and anxiety symptoms and disorders, reductions in existing symptoms of depression, anxiety and distress, and enhanced feelings of well-being."

If you're someone who is feeling depressed or anxious, please consider exercise as a way of improving how you feel. If you experience mood swings, exercise is also for you. I love this quote from Jasper Smits[5], director of the Anxiety Research and Treatment Program at Southern Methodist University in Dallas (USA):

 "A bad mood is no longer a barrier to exercise; it is the very reason to exercise."

By now it's obvious I think that exercise is an important part of your armoury to get you through this time. Research confirms that I'm right. You might think that this isn't enough to make you want to do it. But as with many of the other

recommendations in this book, exercise has many other benefits just waiting for you. Exercise offers you so much more than
just a way to deal with menopausal symptoms.

Even if you've never exercised before, you can start and
experience the benefits. A study[6] of 234 Spanish postmenopausal women aged 45 to 64 years who had at least 12
months of sedentary behaviour should give you hope.

The participants took part in a supervised 20-week exercise
program. After the intervention, the participants experienced
positive changes in short and long-term physical and mental
health, including significant improvements in their cardiovascular fitness and flexibility. But that wasn't all, the participants
achieved modest but significant reductions in their weight and
body mass index. Their hot flashes were also managed better.

Many women overestimate the amount of exercise they
need to take to prevent weight gain. If you think you are going
to have to exercise a lot like a lot of influencers do, you may
decide to do nothing. Yet research suggests you don't have to
exercise obsessively to experience the benefits. And here's a
great quote:

 *"Exercise is a celebration of what your body can do. Not
a punishment for what you ate." Kevin Ng*

EXERCISE & MUSCLE MASS

As women transition from perimenopause to post-menopause
the production of oestrogen reduces dramatically. Reduction in
oestrogen has an effect on muscles and leads to a decline in
muscle mass. Reduction in muscle mass means you are less
strong. This can really affect your confidence. This can lead to
fragility and anxiety, which often means older women want to
stay close to home because of a fear of falling. A reduction in
muscle mass also means that your posture is likely to get worse,

possibly making you seem older than you are. It also means you are more prone to injury.

A reduction in muscle mass also means you are likely to gain weight. The body uses more calories to maintain muscle than it does fat. If you have less muscle mass, you will need fewer calories. But most people don't make that reduction. So, they gradually put on weight. Exercise also tones your body, so that you look better.

Fortunately, physical activity in all of its forms may help maintain muscle mass in midlife.

A study[7] of over a thousand women between the ages of 47 and 55 found that physical activity was positively associated with the maintenance of muscle mass during the menopausal transition. Women who were more active had higher muscle mass before and after menopause compared to the less active women. It seems that even though menopause alone decreases muscle mass, staying physically active throughout middle age can help women to slow the change.

And remember that muscle at rest weighs more than fat at rest. Even a slight increase in muscle mass will mean that your body will need more calories to maintain itself even when you are watching a film or fast asleep in bed.

Many women are fearful of becoming too muscular. This is not a problem for most young women and is certainly not a problem for women in their forties and older. Retaining muscle mass means your posture will be better. You'll be stronger. Your body will be more toned and you will be less likely to injure yourself.

HOW TO MOTIVATE YOURSELF TO EXERCISE

Influencers often talk about getting motivated to exercise and setting goals, but there's a fair amount of research that suggests that focussing on motivation is not the total solution it's often thought to be.

The World Cancer Research Fund[8] says:

"Motivation is temporary and on a rainy Monday in the middle of winter, you'll likely forget what having motivation even feels like. So instead build a small daily habit that in time will become routine, such as 20 minutes of yoga before breakfast or a walk to work in the morning to avoid the rush-hour traffic."

If you talk to most long-term exercisers, they are people who don't so much focus on motivation, as focus on habit with exercise being a priority habit. Long term exercisers don't book a hair appointment and then realise it clashes with the Pilates class that they were intending to go to. Long-term exercisers don't organise a boozy dinner the day before they are planning to run a half marathon. Long-term exercisers have any kit they need washed and within easy reach. Long-term exercisers focus on doing it rather than not doing it. They recognise that there will be some days when they don't feel like exercising, but they will still do it, unless they are ill.

Get the idea? Long-term exercisers have an attitude where exercise is an important part of their lives, without indecision or drama.

They usually have a bigger focus than weight loss and looking good. Of course, that might be part of it. I love going to the gym and lifting weights. I do it consistently week in and week out. My focus is on improving how I function – improving balance, flexibility and co-ordination as well as strength. Other long-term exercisers may be focussing on running faster or being able to do some particular yoga poses better.

Find a form of exercise you enjoy and make it part of your daily life, not just an add-on when you are fed up with feeling fat or before a holiday.

EXERCISE SNACKING

If you haven't done any exercise for a long time, you may be nervous about starting. A way to ease yourself into it is with exercise snacking. This is also great if you can't find the time to exercise.

Exercise snacking, as its name suggests, involves doing exercises through the day in short bursts. We all know that food snacking is fun, but it does, of course, come with a downside of weight gain. Exercise snacking can also be fun, and it, of course, comes with numerous health benefits.

Exercise snacking can lead to you wanting to take more exercise, maybe go to a class, join the gym or start running.

Here are some suggestions of things you could do. It's best if you can attach them to some other activity that you always do during the day. That way you are much more likely to remember to do them.

Stand on one leg while you clean your teeth in the morning. In the evening stand on the other leg while you clean your teeth. You do clean your teeth twice a day, don't you?

Dawn Skelton[9], Professor in Ageing and Health, Glasgow Caledonian University, writes

"Research shows that people's ability to stand on one leg is an indicator of health and that getting better at standing on one leg can add to fitness and potentially lifespan.

"Being able to stand on one leg is linked to increased levels of physical activity and decreased risk of falls and is associated with both quality and length of life."

She goes on to say that you can improve your ability to balance on one leg regardless of how old you are.

Another possibility is to do air squats while talking on the phone. Air squats are also known as body weight squats. Here's how to do them:

- Keep your feet pointed straight ahead, shoulder width apart.
- Keep your back straight, don't round your shoulders.
- Keep your eyes on something ahead of you and your chest lifted.
- Push your butt back and bend your knees.
- Your knee shouldn't be further forward than your toes.
- Concentrate on "sitting" between your legs to minimise leaning forward.
- Go as low as you can, while keeping your whole foot on the floor.

Run up and down the stairs for 4 minutes three times a day. Attach this to a meal, (preferably before the meal!), to help you remember to do it. To start with running may be out of the question, so you may have to settle for walking briskly.

A study reported by Washington University[10] found that just a few minutes of stair climbing dispersed throughout the day had measurable impact on heart health.

For the study, each "exercise snack" involved going up a three-flight staircase one step at a time, as quickly as possible. Each "snack" was preceded by a warm-up of 10 jumping jacks, 10 air squats and five lunges on each side, and followed by a cool-down of 1 minute of level walking.

By performing this activity three times a day (with 1 to 4 hours of rest in-between) three days of the week over a six-week period, study participants improved their maximal oxygen uptake — a measurement of cardiovascular fitness.

If that sounds too difficult, put it on one side for the time being, but revisit it as you get fitter. Try this instead. Touch your toes (or as near as you can get), while emptying your dishwasher:

- Touch your toes three times
- Take out a set of plates and put them away
- Touch your toes three times
- Take out more crockery or cutlery
- Repeat until the dishwasher is empty

Another possibility is to bring in your shopping and then use the weight of your shopping bag to do a suitcase carry: You simply carry the shopping bag in one hand and walk around with it. Engage your core (your abdominal muscles). Keep your shoulders level and facing forward. If you have to lean over to one side to carry the shopping, the bag is too heavy. Put some of the shopping away and carry a lighter weight. You will improve and eventually amaze yourself at the weights you can lift.

Want something more difficult? Do" round the clocks" while the kettle boils. There are various ways of doing this, but this is the way I do it:

- I brace my core and stand on one leg, imaging that I'm standing inside a clock face that is on the ground.
- I touch the other foot lightly on the 12 o'clock position in front of me.
- Then I touch 3 o'clock to the right of me.
- Then I touch the foot behind me to the 6 o'clock position.
- Then I bring the leg round to the front and over to the left side and touch the 9 o'clock position. (Sometimes I touch the 9 o'clock position from behind and then from the front! Is that showing off?)

Then I repeat with the other foot. I try to make sure that the moving foot touches as lightly as possible, without any weight. If you find this difficult at first, let your foot rest more heavily at each clock position. You may need to hold a works surface when you first start, but if you keep doing it, you will progress and delight yourself.

These are a few ideas for exercise snacking, but I'm sure you can think of more for yourself now that you get the idea.

WHAT DO YOU DO WHEN YOU HATE EXERCISE?

I was talking to a friend in her sixties, who told me she hates exercise. She knows she should do it but hates it. She said it almost as though that settled the matter. She didn't need to do any, because she hated it.

Now that approach may be OK for not reading Tolstoy or not eating bananas, but it's really not OK when it comes to exercise and some other daily activities.

What would she have said to me if I'd said: "I hate cleaning my teeth, so I don't do it."

I think she would have been shocked. She would have thought that it didn't matter that I hated it. I still absolutely needed to clean my teeth to avoid bad breath and to prevent dental caries. She might have even told me that. And, of course, she would have been right.

You really need to view exercise as being a truly important part of your life. It's probably more important, than cleaning your teeth.

The UK NHS used to say on their website that 8 out of 10 people think they exercise enough, but in reality, only 3 out of 10 actually do. I can't find this quote now, but I still imagine there are a lot of people who think they exercise enough even though they don't.

Many people fool themselves that they are doing more than they think, because they hate exercise so much. So, the big questions is: if I hate exercise, how can I make it fun and enjoyable?

There some obvious things to try: exercise snacking, working out with a friend, joining a class, trying something new, etc. But what if you still hate it? Then your approach needs to be: I hate exercise. I'm always going to hate it, but I'm going to do it.

So, you could treat exercise as a necessary evil. It's something you need to do to keep your body and mind toned and strong. You might surprise yourself and develop a taste for it after all.

I find the best way of dealing with unpleasant things that I need to do is to work out how much the time is as a proportion of my life.

For example, I'm in my seventies, so I'm going to assume for this calculation that I will live to be 90.

90 years = 47,304,000 minutes

You can see what a small part of my life the current 30-minute workout would be (I'm not going to give you some impossible fraction here!) I focus on this when I'm doing something unpleasant.

You may want to experiment to find the type of exercise you hate the least! But just accept that you will always hate it, but that you will do it. You will focus on the results you will achieve rather than the time you spend doing the exercise.

And if you hate exercise, don't believe it's OK to reward yourself with a chocolate bar or a doughnut because of the calories you've just used up exercising. People generally overestimate the number of calories they use. Exercise classes will often give the wrong impression of how many calories you'll burn – up to 800 calories, doesn't mean that's what you'll burn.

Maria Brilaki[11] says:

"If you have to force yourself to do it, then there is a 90% chance that you are doing it wrong and you will never stick to exercise."

She then goes on to suggest strategies to help yourself to take exercise. Yet some people are never going to enjoy any form of exercise. But (like cleaning your teeth) that doesn't mean you don't do it.

Stop chasing that perennial question of how to enjoy exercise when you hate it, and just do it. This is the "feel the hate and do it anyway" approach to exercise!

You may want to exercise but feel you shouldn't because of some health condition, so let's take a look at that.

SHOULD I EXERCISE IF I HAVE BACK PAIN?

It's not so long ago that you would have been advised by your doctor to rest if you had back pain, but that advice has changed in the face of mounting evidence. Now health authorities are happy to encourage you to stay as active as you possibly can.

This, for example, is the advice of the NHS[12]:

"One of the most important things you can do is to keep moving and continue with your normal activities as much as possible.

"It used to be thought that bed rest would help you recover from a bad back, but it's now known that people who remain active are likely to recover quicker.

"This may be difficult at first, but do not be discouraged – your pain should start to improve eventually."

The WebMD[13] agrees:

"You may feel like resting, but moving is good for your back. Exercises for lower back pain can strengthen back, stomach, and leg muscles. They help support your spine, relieving back pain."

Jatinder Gill, MD[14], an anesthesiologist and back pain specialist at BIDMC's William Arnold – Carol A. Warfield, MD Pain Center (USA) says:

"Unless there are serious red flags – pain shooting down to your legs or incontinence – my first recommendation is to remain fully active ... The best thing you can do is try to move on. Too much resting and lying down are not good for your back.

"Through a process called neuroadaptation, the body can adjust to pain, and the pain dissipates ... Remaining active despite some aches and pains is a very powerful tool in creating this neuroadaptation."

The authorities are agreed that exercising can help back pain. Of course, if you're used to using heavy weights in the gym, you may need to use lighter weights, rest more between sets and do fewer reps. If you're a runner, you may need to run less fast or for a shorter time.

The website relaxtheback.com[15] explains

"Back pain workouts help you recover from back pain, strengthen weak muscles and increase flexibility in tight areas. Over the years, several studies have found that physical activity decreases self-reported pain symptoms, not just for low back pain but for osteoporosis and arthritis as well. Research also shows that weight-training programs improve short-term and long-term pain symptoms.

"Weak back muscles fail to help the spine carry its load, putting unnecessary pressure on spinal discs. That's why maintaining strong back and core muscles is so essential for preventing back pain."

The general recommendation is to exercise even if you have back pain, but there are some situations where you shouldn't. The US Mayo Clinic[16] says:

"Call your doctor if your back pain hasn't improved after a week of home treatment or if your back pain:

- Is constant or intense, especially at night or when you lie down
- Spreads down one or both legs, especially if the pain extends below your knee

- Causes weakness, numbness or tingling in one or both legs
- Occurs with unintended weight loss
- Occurs with swelling or redness on your back

Scott Weiss[17], a New York physical therapist and athletic trainer offers more detailed advice. He says there are some instances when it's smarter to go to your doctor rather than go to the gym. These include:

- If the pain worsens at night and while lying flat
- if it persists for six weeks or more
- if it's associated with weight loss and fever
- if you've recently fallen
- if you have osteoporosis
- if you have shooting pain down one or both legs
- if you have suddenly crooked posture
- if you cannot stand up straight
- if you have to hold your breath when changing position

You may be glad to understand that returning to exercising is beneficial for your back most of the time. But is it safe to exercise if you have back pain and have never exercised? Of course, it's best to get medical advice on this and start slowly.

Walking can be a great place to start, gradually increasing the number of steps you take each day. If possible, use a pedometer or smart watch to monitor your progress and encourage you to do more. Walking briskly and other exercises stimulate endorphins, which naturally reduce your sensations of pain.

Doing stretching and strengthening exercises can really help back pain. Check out the HASfit website[18] for videos of exercise routines you can do at home. It's all free and they have specific ones for back pain.

SHOULD I EXERCISE IF I HAVE CANCER OR HAVE HAD CANCER?

We know that physical exercise is an important part of preventing chronic diseases. The CDC (USA) puts it clearly[19]:

"Regular physical activity helps improve your overall health, fitness, and quality of life. It also helps reduce your risk of chronic conditions like type 2 diabetes, heart disease, many types of cancer, depression and anxiety, and dementia."

Reviewing the existing research on cancer prevention and exercise, University of British Columbia (Canada) researchers[20] say:

"For all adults, exercise is important for cancer prevention and specifically lowers risk of seven common types of cancer: colon, breast, endometrial, kidney, bladder, esophagus and stomach."

But can exercise help you if you already have cancer or are recovering from cancer?

I fully agree with what cancer.net[21] says:

"Always talk with your doctor before you start an exercise program during or after cancer treatment. While exercise is proven to be safe during different types of cancer treatment, your ability to exercise and the types of exercises you can do depends on:

- The type of cancer you have
- The treatments being used
- The side effects that you are experiencing
- Your level of fitness
- Your other health problems"

The American Cancer Society[22] gives very clear advice:

"In the past, people being treated for a chronic illness (an illness a person may live with for a long time, like cancer or diabetes) were often told by their doctor to rest and reduce their physical activity. This is good advice if movement causes pain, rapid heart rate, or shortness of breath. But newer research has shown that exercise is not only safe and possible during cancer treatment, but it can improve how well you function physically and your quality of life.

"Too much rest can lead to loss of body function, muscle weakness, and reduced range of motion. So today, many cancer care teams are urging their patients to be as physically active as possible during cancer treatment. Many people are learning about the advantages of being physically active after treatment, too."

Cancer.net[23] agrees with this advice:

"Exercise is an important part of a cancer treatment plan. A growing amount of research shows that regular exercise can greatly improve physical and mental health during every phase of treatment. Even if you were not active before your cancer diagnosis, an exercise program that meets your unique needs can help you get moving safely and successfully."

The Dana-Faber Cancer Institute[24] (USA) says:

"Exercising, even at a moderate level, is one thing cancer survivors can do to lower the odds of cancer recurrence. The most consistent and largest number of studies looking at the links between exercise and cancer recurrence and overall survival have been reported for patients with breast and colorectal cancer, though increasingly other cancer types are also being studied."

University of British Columbia[25] (Canada) researchers are also clear about this:

"For the rising number of cancer survivors worldwide,

there's growing evidence that exercise is an important part of recovery.

"For cancer survivors, incorporate exercise to help improve survival after a diagnosis of breast, colon and prostate cancer.

"Exercising during and after cancer treatment improves fatigue, anxiety, depression, physical function, quality of life and does not exacerbate lymphedema."

This last sentence is particularly interesting. Exercise **reduces** the fatigue associated with many cancer treatments. This is counter-intuitive but well proven by the research.

The Australian Cancer Council[26] says this about cancer fatigue and exercise:

"Feeling tired, even when rested, is common in people with cancer. Sometimes it lasts for months after treatment ends. Staying active can help ease fatigue. Try adjusting how hard and how often you exercise – some people find shorter, frequent aerobic sessions are more manageable; others prefer strength-based training. Losing fitness and strength can make fatigue worse. Doing some low intensity exercise can help you maintain your fitness and strength (unless you have severe anaemia)."

The Mayo Clinic[27] points to the psychological feelings that you are doing something and not just being "done to":

"The evidence keeps rolling in: Exercise can be one of your most important cancer treatments. For anyone dealing with a cancer diagnosis, that's great news. Starting - or maintaining - an exercise program can empower you to move out of a more passive "patient" role; it'll help improve not just your well-being but your attitude, too."

Have you got the message? Exercise is important as a cancer prevention strategy, and it's likely to help if you are in the middle of cancer treatment.

I've spent some time on this not because hormonal changes cause cancers, but because the incidence of some cancers increases around this time as a result of aging. I don't want you to think exercise isn't for you because of cancer.

SHOULD I EXERCISE IF I HAVE OSTEOPOROSIS?

Exercise can help prevent osteoporosis (see the chapter on Osteoporosis), but what about people who are at a high risk of osteoporotic fractures or have a formal diagnosis of osteoporosis? It's an important question because it's estimated that 137 million women and 21 million men have high osteoporotic fracture risk globally. Fractures can lead to long-term pain, loss of independence, disability and reduced life expectancy.

In 2022 a UK multi-disciplinary panel of experts[28] reviewed existing evidence and drew on clinical and patient opinion to reach agreement on recommendations to maximise bone health while minimising fracture risk. This consensus statement was endorsed by the Royal Osteoporosis Society (UK). The panel summarised their view:

"There is little evidence that physical activity is associated with significant harm, and the benefits, in general, outweigh the risks."

I am going to quote their specific recommendations at length, because I think it's important to see how they really are recommending exercise for people in all stages of osteoporosis. The intensity of the exercise will vary, but even those with fractures are recommended to exercise.

For all people with osteoporosis:

- Muscle-strengthening physical activity and exercise is recommended on two or three days of the week to maintain bone strength.
- For maximum benefit, muscle strengthening should include progressive muscle resistance training. In practice, this is the maximum that can be lifted 8–12

times (building up to three sets for each exercise). Lower intensity exercise ensuring good technique is recommended before increasing intensity levels.

- All muscle groups should be targeted, including back muscles to promote bone strength in the spine.
- Daily physical activity is recommended as a minimum, spread across the day and avoiding prolonged periods of sitting.

In addition:

For people with osteoporosis who do not have vertebral fractures or multiple low-trauma fractures:

- Moderate impact exercise is recommended on most days to promote bone strength (eg, stamping, jogging, low-level jumping, hopping) to include at least 50 impacts per session (jogs, hops etc).
- Brief bursts of moderate impact physical activity should be considered: about 50 impacts (eg, 5 sets of 10) with reduced impact in between (eg, walk-jog).

For people with osteoporosis who have vertebral fractures or multiple low trauma fractures:

- Impact exercise on most days at a level up to brisk walking is recommended, aiming for 150 minutes over the week (20 min per day). This a precautionary measure because of theoretical (unproved) risks of further vertebral fracture in this group.
- Individualised advice from a physiotherapist is recommended for both impact and progressive resistance training to ensure correct technique, at least at the start of a new programme of exercise or activity.

For people with osteoporosis who are frail and/or less able to exercise:

- Physical activity and exercise to help maintain bone strength should be adapted according to individual ability.
- Strength and balance exercise to prevent falls will be needed for confidence and stability before physical activity levels are increased. In practice, falls prevention may be a priority.

The conclusion from this panel of experts is clear: even if you have osteoporosis, you should be exercising daily.

IS SHAME STOPPING YOU EXERCISING?

Are you intimidated by the idea of going to the gym or starting to run? Do you feel people would laugh at you if you went to a yoga class? Or do you feel you need to get fit before you start publicly exercising?

Recently I got talking to an overweight lady in our gym. She hadn't been coming for long, so I asked her how she was enjoying it. She told me she found it very hard work. I told her that if she wanted to make progress, it was always going to be hard work, because you'll keep on wanting to improve.

She then started to talk about "body shaming" and how difficult it had been to start coming to the gym. I told her that most people were so engrossed in what they were doing, they weren't paying her any attention.

I also said that many people seem to feel they must have a gym body BEFORE they go to the gym. Of course, the way you get a gym body is by going to the gym and working out. But many people have a fear of being ridiculed at the gym. They have a sort of fantasy that they will lose weight and get toned or strong in the secrecy of their own home. Then they will already look amazing when they finally go to the gym. They have never managed to do this, but the fantasy persists.

She nodded and laughed. But she said a bigger problem for her was her own sense of shame in her body.

I remember reading about a woman who wanted to start running. She was very overweight. She felt that people would laugh at her if she started running. To begin with she ran in a coat and with a shopping bag, so that people would just think she was running to the shops. Once she had reached a level of speed and fitness, she ditched the coat and the shopping bag. This made me laugh at the time, but I was also impressed at her ingenuity in finding a solution that allowed her to get fit without feeling overcome by embarrassment. I'm not saying you should do this, but if a strategy like this will allow you to start exercising, go for it!

I learnt to ride a bike when I was in my forties. My partner was keen to encourage me, so he wanted to buy me the latest kit. He thought he was encouraging me. I found it so difficult. I felt that people would laugh at me because I wasn't "really" a cyclist. I wasn't fast enough or confident enough or thin enough. Only real cyclists could or should wear the latest lycra cycling clothes or have an expensive cycling helmet. Fortunately, it didn't stop me riding my bike and getting faster, more confident and fitter. Eventually I was happy to wear the latest kit. One day I realised I'd prefer a new pair of cycling shorts to a dress. At that point I realised I must be a real cyclist.

The woman I met in the gym recently is going despite her sense of shame. She told me she tells herself repeatedly that she is doing something about it, and that is what counts. That keeps her coming. I have so much admiration for this woman and her attitude.

Naomi Teeter describes herself as a "Health coach, weight

loss expert, and former plus-sizer." In a Huffington Post article[29] she writes:

"Do you have the need to look capable at all times? Do you try not to work too hard in front of others (exerting effort, sweating, etc.)? When faced with a setback, do you hide your flaws or avoid the situation entirely? Does it seem pointless to even try? If you resonated with any of these questions, you might be too embarrassed to exercise in front of others due to a perfectionistic, fixed mindset."

She goes on to write:

"It may not be clear when this mindset originated, but at some point, it became your truth that natural born physical (and mental) ability is far superior to trying (and struggling)."

Naomi recommends developing a growth mindset rather than a perfectionist mindset. This will allow you to go to the gym and do things imperfectly.

Working with a personal trainer can help you overcome your feeling of shame. Going to the gym or an exercise class with a friend can help. Being prepared to be uncomfortable because you keep your big plan in mind – to live a healthy life – can help too.

Don't let your sense of shame interfere with your desire to get fitter. Working out, getting strong and toned will help you feel better about yourself. Overcoming your sense of shame and going despite how you feel about yourself is a real triumph for your determination and strength of character.

Shame is such a damaging emotion. Social media makes this worse for many young people. We older women have a duty to overcome the shame that stops us exercising. If we can't do it, how can we expect our daughters and granddaughters to do it?

And you never know, you could inspire others. I'm in my seventies and go to the gym regularly. Young people often tell me I'm inspirational. Several have said that when they see their parents, they are downhearted about what happens to your body when you get older. Seeing me working out and functioning well gives them reassurance that it can be different. Start exercising – not only could you end up a lot healthier, but you could inspire others. How amazing would that be?

Here's a quote to inspire you:

 "To escape criticism – do nothing, say nothing, be nothing" Elbert Hubbard

WHAT EXERCISE SHOULD I DO?

The bottom line is that you should probably do more than you are doing now. Just get started. Try to find something you enjoy, but you also need to see some progress. You will only see progress if you put effort into it. Sadly, many women see exercise as mainly a social event, and a chance to eat cake without feeling guilty!

If you see exercise as a social event, you are likely to be so busy talking that you won't be concentrating on the workout you are supposed to be doing. This means that you won't be working out hard enough. If you're not working out hard enough, you won't see any improvement. If you don't see any improvement, you might as well cut out the exercise and move straight to the cake!

Over and over again I see women eating lots of calories after they've been for a brisk walk or to an exercise class on the grounds that they've just burnt a lot of calories. If you've worked out hard, you do need to refuel afterwards, but the food you eat should be nutritious not just high calorie.

If you are deciding what type of activity to do, here are some suggestions. I've included specific information about them, because the research shows they are beneficial for women at this time.

RESISTANCE EXERCISES/STRENGTH TRAINING

Resistance training (also called weight training and strength training) is so beneficial for women of your age. The gyms are full of young women lifting weights, but the benefit to women of your age is much much bigger.

The Association of UK Dietitians[30] says:

"Resistance activities, such as using weights, are especially important to both preserve and build muscle mass."

Research published in the academic journal BMC Musculoskeletal Disorders[31] concluded:

"The overall findings suggest that exercise may result in clinically relevant benefits to … BMD [bone mineral density] in postmenopausal women."

The UC San Diego School of Medicine[32] (USA) puts it clearly:

"Strength training has a multitude of benefits for chronic disease management. With consistent strength training, patients with arthritis showed decreased pain, individuals with Type-2 diabetes showed improved glucose control, and the increase in bone mineral density helps manage and prevent osteoporosis."

Many women are frightened of injuring themselves with resistance training. The same website says this:

"By strengthening bones and muscles through strength training, your body can build a higher resistance to injuries, aches, and pains as well as reduce the severity of falls."

Personally, I know this to be true. Before I started resistance training, I used to have sciatic pain from time to time. Now I don't. I'm always in a hurry and in my impatience have had some horrible falls. But I recover easily and don't break any bones. I used to get low back pain if I had to stand for long. Now it only happens if I'm standing for a really long time.

Many older women worry about dementia. The good news is that researchers at the University of Sydney[33] have shown that strength training in older people protects some regions of the brain from shrinkage. They believe that lifting weights should be a standard part of dementia reduction programmes.

Janet Viljoen[34], a research fellow in physical activity and health at Rhodes University (South Africa) looked at the benefits of strength training for a group of women aged 55 to 65.

The women exercised in small groups with a personal trainer for two months. They did exercises that targeted their upper bodies, torsos and legs for 30 minutes, five times a week. The programme got progressively harder as the women progressed.

The results were extremely encouraging. The women built up strength in both their upper and lower bodies. They were also more confident and happier. For many women increasing confidence around this time is a huge bonus. In general, they didn't lose any weight, but that wasn't the purpose of the study.

The women also found improvements in their everyday lives – climbing stairs, getting up and down from the floor and playing with grandchildren were all easier because of the strength training. They also had less knee and hip pain.

She concludes her article with:

"The good news is that strength training can have tangible outcomes. Many women give up on less intense exercise programmes, like walking, because they feel there is no benefit. Now they know they have an alternative."

It's really important to make sure you are always challenging yourself. Often women tell me the gym is boring or it doesn't work. I think this is often because when they go to the gym, they don't challenge themselves. I've seen women chatting to friends while lifting dumbbells with ease. I've seen women walking on treadmill at a pace slower than they walk upstairs. If this is what you do, I can tell you categorically that you won't see any improvement. You will get bored and decide it doesn't work. If you challenge yourself and see improvement, you will be amazed at the difference it makes to your life generally. You will be motivated to do more exercise.

I may have convinced you about the benefits of resistance training, but you still might not want to go to the gym. You may not be able to go, because of family commitments or financial barriers.

If you'd rather exercise at home, take a look at the HASfit website[35]. This website has lots of free workouts you can do at home. You don't need equipment for some of the workouts, but for others you will need one pair of dumbbells, or you could use water bottles. The site offers workouts of various lengths. They have workouts you can do sitting down, low impact workouts, ones to create muscle or burn fat. There are stretching routines and so much more. They are all free. I highly recommend this website.

TAI CHI

Tai chi originates in ancient China. It involves a series of gentle physical exercises and stretches in a set order. Each posture flows into the next, so that the body is constantly moving at a slow pace. Tai chi has been described as "meditation in motion". It's vastly different from a Zumba class or a run.

Harvard Medical School[36] enthusiastically endorses tai chi for everyone:

"Although tai chi is slow and gentle and doesn't leave you breathless, it addresses the key components of fitness — muscle strength, flexibility, balance, and, to a lesser degree, aerobic conditioning."

Tai chi may be beneficial for menopausal symptoms, but there isn't clear evidence that this is so. A review in the journal Osteoporosis International[37] concluded:

"Tai chi exercise may have benefits on bone health in perimenopausal and postmenopausal women, but the evidence is sometimes weak, poor, and inconsistent."

This doesn't mean that tai chi won't help you. It simply means that the evidence isn't there to say with confidence that it's helpful for many menopausal women. There are other studies that conclude that tai chi is beneficial for the problems many women experience during menopausal transition and later in their lives.

A study in the Journal of Aging Research[38] found that:

"Tai Chi would be a good physical activity design for aged women in order to increase their antioxidant protection and to prevent oxidative stress-related metabolic diseases [such as type 2 diabetes and cardiovascular disease]."

Tai chi has also been found to be beneficial for other age-related problems. In a study published in the Journal of Rheumatology[39] 72 women with osteoarthritis were randomly put into an experimental or control group. They completed pre and post-test measures over 12 weeks. Results show the Tai Chi group ended up with 35% less pain, 29% less stiffness, 29% higher ability to perform daily tasks (like climbing stairs), improved abdominal muscles and better balance.

Other studies have shown that tai chi can be beneficial for back pain and fall prevention. A small feasibility study published by the European Society of Cardiology[40] has suggested that tai chi has the potential to reduce depression, anxiety and stress plus improve sleep in people who have had a stroke. This doesn't mean it will work for menopausal and post-menopausal women who have these symptoms, but it's certainly worth trying.

YOGA

Yoga has been shown to be beneficial for weight management for people of all ages (see Hack 129 in my book "190 Weight

Loss Hacks: What The Evidence Says"). In particular it seems to encourage regular yoga participants to follow a healthier lifestyle. Many participants value the sense of friendship in their yoga group, so this could be a good strategy for you if you feel short of good friends. But there is more specific research showing that it's beneficial for menopausal women too.

Márcia P. Jorge and colleagues published an article in Complementary Therapies in Medicine[41], looking at the benefits of hatha yoga for menopausal symptoms. 88 post-menopausal women volunteered for this 12-week trial. They were randomly assigned to one of three groups: control (no intervention), exercise, and yoga.

After 12 weeks those practising yoga had statistically lower scores for menopausal symptoms, stress levels and depression symptoms, as well as significantly higher scores in quality of life when compared to control and exercise groups.

Another study[42] of integral yoga found that women in the yoga group reported a decrease of approximately 66% in hot flash frequency.

All this suggests it's well worth trying yoga. Many women find it enjoyable for its own sake and some find a community of like-minded women for support and friendship.

The National Institute of Health[43] (USA) says:

"There's … evidence that yoga may be helpful for some medical conditions. Yoga may help lessen pain and menopause symptoms."

DANCE

If you have a lingering hatred of sport and exercise from your school days, what about trying dance? When you think about exercising, you may not think about dance.

A study published in *Menopause*, the journal of The North American Menopause Society[44] found that a dance class three times a week improved not only fitness and metabolic profile but also self-image and self-esteem in postmenopausal women.

COLD-WATER SWIMMING/WILD SWIMMING

Cold-water swimming has become popular in recent years, and many older women say it's beneficial. The BBC[45] reported that a group of women in Wales has said that plunging into sea temperatures as cold as 6C was helping with menopausal symptoms. Some women also reported improvements in their mental health. Professor Mike Tipton, an expert in cold water swimming at the University of Portsmouth (UK) says there's lots of anecdotal evidence about the value of cold-water swimming. He goes on to say that most cold-water swimmers do it with groups of other people, so some of the benefit that swimmers report could be down to the social element as well as the actual experience of the cold water.

If you want to try cold-water swimming, please make sure you start with a group of people who know what they are doing. Don't just plunge into a cold lake or sea and hope for the best.

INSOMNIA/SLEEP

*M*aybe you've never slept well or maybe night sweats and anxiety are keeping you awake as you go through the hormonal changes associated with this time.

When you fall asleep, your brain is not merely offline, it's busy organizing new memories. If you don't get enough sleep, this process doesn't happen properly. During sleep, the brain replays neural firing patterns experienced while awake, also known as "offline replay." Replay is thought to underlie memory consolidation, the process by which recent memories acquire more permanence in their neural representation. Sleep disturbances interfere with this important process.

Lack of sleep can also affect your mood. You probably already know that! Researchers from the University of British Columbia[1] (Canada) found that after a night of shorter sleep, people react more emotionally to stressful events the next day. They don't find as much joy in the good things. This has important health implications: previous research shows that being unable to maintain positive emotions in the face of stress puts people at risk of inflammation and even an earlier death.

Research[2] published in the American Heart Association's

flagship journal *Circulation* found that after adjusting for diabetes, hypertension, medication use, genetic variations and other covariates, participants with the healthiest sleep pattern had a 42% reduction in the risk of heart failure compared to people with an unhealthy sleep pattern.

CAN INSOMNIA CAUSE WEIGHT GAIN?

Disrupted sleep is also likely to increase the possibility of weight gain and make losing weight harder. Researchers Emma Sweeney (Lecturer in Exercise and Health, Nottingham Trent University, UK) and Ian Walshe (Lecturer in Health and Exercise Sciences, Northumbria University, Newcastle) write[3]:

"Sleep influences two important appetite hormones in our body – leptin and ghrelin. Leptin is a hormone that decreases appetite, so when leptin levels are high we usually feel fuller. On the other hand, ghrelin is a hormone that can stimulate appetite, and is often referred to as the "hunger hormone" because it's thought to be responsible for the feeling of hunger."

Dr. Michael Twery, a sleep expert at the National Institute of Health[4] (USA) says:

"Sleep affects almost every tissue in our bodies ... It affects growth and stress hormones, our immune system, appetite, breathing, blood pressure and cardiovascular health. Ongoing research shows a lack of sleep can produce diabetic-like conditions in otherwise healthy people."

MENOPAUSAL SLEEP DISTURBANCE

The North American Menopause Society recognises that some women find they experience sleep disturbances during menopause. These are often attributed to menopause, but the Society says[5]:

" ... there are many reasons for sleep disturbances besides

menopausal night sweats (simply, hot flashes at night). Your sleep disturbances may be caused by factors that affect many women beginning at midlife, such as sleep-disordered breathing (known as sleep apnea), restless legs syndrome, stress, anxiety, depression, painful chronic illnesses, and even some medications."

Enrica Bonnani and colleagues from the University of Pisa[6] (Italy) write:

"The medical conditions that may compromise sleep in this age group [menopausal women] are common; they include obesity, gastroesophageal reflux, cancer, urinary incontinence and nocturia, thyroid dysfunction, chronic pain, fibromyalgia (often starting or worsening in menopause), and hypertension. Common causes of sleep disorders in middle-aged women include poor sleep hygiene, volitional factors, environmental disturbances, alcohol intake, marital dissatisfaction, requests for care from children, grandchildren and/or elderly parents, and financial worries."

In other words, don't automatically assume that your sleep disturbance is caused by hormonal changes. I hope this sounds familiar now. We also found that for weight gain.

A study by researchers[7] from the University of Pennsylvania (USA) and Johns Hopkins University (USA) concluded:

"Clinicians can expect that many mid-life women report sleep difficulties. However, clinicians should consider that poor sleep is not simply due to menopause or hot flashes, given the evidence that premenopausal sleep status was the strongest predictor of poor sleep in the menopause transition. Hot flashes were strongly associated with poor sleep as expected, but a large proportion of poor sleep in the menopause transition occurred *without* hot flashes."

If you're faced with insomnia or other problems, it may feel easier to blame your hormones rather than look at other factors such as alcohol intake, marital dissatisfaction or long-term poor sleep habits. Yet, if you ignore these factors, the long-term health implications will be significant.

MAKING SLEEP A PRIORITY

It's easy to think of sleep as being something that happens when you run out of things to do or you can no longer keep your eyes open. Dr. Kara Duraccio[8] of Brigham Young University (USA) says:

"It's human nature to think that when we have a long to-do list, sleep should be the first thing to go or the easiest thing to cut out ... We don't recognize that getting enough sleep helps you accomplish your to-do list better."

It's really important to get enough sleep if you want to lose or maintain your weight. If you want to be happy and enjoy life, sleep is important. If you want to be healthy, sleep has to be a high priority.

Value sleep for what it gives you in many different aspects of your life.

REDUCE HOT FLASHES/NIGHT SWEATS

One of the most important things many women can do is find ways of reducing the number of hot flashes and night sweats they experience. Check out Chapter XX to find out how to do this.

SET REGULAR HOURS

The UK NHS[9] advises:

"First of all, keep regular sleeping hours. This programmes the brain and internal body clock to get used to a set routine."

Obviously, there will be days when this is not possible, but there will be many days when you can do this. It may need some planning and involving other members of your household. You will be doing them a favour if in supporting you it encourages them to set regular hours too.

REDUCE BLUE LIGHT

Curlicue compact fluorescent lightbulbs and LED lights are better for the environment, but unfortunately have health implications for us because of the amount of blue light they emit.

Harvard Health Publishing[10] offers the following advice:

- "Use dim red lights for night lights. Red light is less likely to shift circadian rhythm and suppress melatonin.
- "Avoid looking at bright screens beginning two to three hours before bed.
- "If you work a night shift or use a lot of electronic devices at night, consider wearing blue-blocking glasses or installing an app that filters the blue/green wavelength at night.
- "Expose yourself to lots of bright light during the day, which will boost your ability to sleep at night, as well as your mood and alertness during daylight."

REDUCE LIGHTING WHILE SLEEPING

A study published in *JAMA Internal Medicine*[11] found that women who slept with some artificial light were more likely to gain weight and develop obesity. The light could be from a television that had been left on, a night light, a mobile phone or streetlights. The study lasted for six years.

The researchers found that women who slept with a light or television on were more likely to be obese at the start of the study. They were also 17% more likely to have gained around 11 pounds (4.9 kg) or more over the follow-up period. The association with light coming from outside the room was more modest. Using a small nightlight wasn't associated with any more weight gain than sleeping with no light.

The authors couldn't rule out all the other factors that might be linked with artificial light at night and weight gain. However, their findings didn't significantly change when they adjusted for age, having an older spouse or children in the home, race, socioeconomic status, where they lived, calories consumed, night-time snacking, physical activity, and sleep length and quality.

A BATH BEFORE BED

Researchers from the University of Texas[12] (USA) found that bathing 1-2 hours before bedtime in water of about 104-109 degrees Fahrenheit (40 - 43 degrees Celsius) can significantly improve your sleep.

TRY MINDFULNESS

There's a lot of interest in mindfulness as an effective self-calming programme in lots of different situations, and I talk in Chapter XX about its use for weight control.

Researchers[13] found that an eight-week mindfulness meditation training programme improved sleep quality, quality of life, attention levels, and reduced hot flashes/night sweats in postmenopausal women with insomnia.

But how do you get enough sleep? Try the Headspace app[14]. This has lots of different tracks to choose from. Try their Sleepcasts series for ever-changing storytelling in a range of soothing voices. The Wind Downs series lead you through meditation and breathing to prepare you for sleep.

Sleep Music gives you calming tracks to help you drift off. If you're in the UK, BBC Sound has a selection of sleep tracks too.

STORIES

Donald Liebell in an article in the Integrative & Complementary Therapies[15] journal says that many people fall asleep while watching television, but when they go to bed they find it difficult to sleep. He says that this is because you are not trying to sleep in front of the TV, but when you go to bed you are trying to sleep. He sees the act of focussing on this goal as getting in the way of relaxing and drifting off to sleep, as happens in front of the television.

He suggests listening to audiobooks:

"Listening to audiobooks provides a distraction from one's own thoughts. It is critical that the listening material does not include commercials, fluctuating volumes, or materials of engagement. The volume should be set at the lowest level possible to clearly listen.

"The intention and mechanism of action is to distract one's mind from active thought, so it can shut down and sleep, naturally. A word of caution: it is critical to never use a cellphone, which is a source of electromagnetic radiation, next to one's head all night. A radiation-free, wire-free, and inexpensive MP3 player with a built-in speaker can go under the pillow and be set to turn off itself in 15–30 minutes."

WORRIES & GRATITUDE

Worries can keep you awake. Avoid looking at or paying bills and similar jobs just before you plan to go to bed.

The Royal College Of Psychiatrists[16] (UK) suggests:

"If something is troubling you and there is nothing you can

do about it right away, try writing it down before going to bed and then tell yourself to deal with it tomorrow."

Also do a simple gratitude process. Before you go to sleep think of three things that have happened (or not happened) in the day and take a moment to name each one and feel grateful for it.

USE ESSENTIAL OILS

Try essential oils, which are widely regarded as having beneficial effects on sleep. There is also now some scientific evidence[17] to support this.

The Royal College Of Psychiatrists[18] (UK) says:

"Take some time to relax properly before going to bed. Some people find aromatherapy helpful."

- Lavender[19] helps slow heart rate and relaxes muscles.
- Sweet marjoram is calming and helps to slow the mind.
- Chamomile and Sandalwood help to reduce anxiety.
- Ylang Ylang has a soothing effect that alleviates stress.
- Peppermint oil[20] aids sleep, probably through reducing stress.

You can use these oils in various ways. For example:

- Put a few drops of oil on a tissue and inhale the vapour
- Add to a carrier oil and then rub on your hands
- Add to water and spray in your room or on your pillow

FLOWER REMEDIES

Try some Bach Flower Remedies (see Chapter XX). You might like to try 'vervain' if you find it difficult to switch off from the day; 'holly' if anger and resentment keep you awake; 'white chestnut' for persistent unwanted thoughts and 'aspen' if you wake because of nightmares.

ALCOHOL

Many people use alcohol to help them sleep, because they feel it helps them get to sleep. But alcohol has been shown to reduce the quality of your sleep.

Drinkaware.co.uk[21] says:

"Regularly drinking alcohol can disrupt sleep. For example, a heavy drinking session of more than six units in an evening, can make us spend more time in deep sleep and less time than usual in the important Rapid Eye Movement (REM) stage of sleep, which is an important restorative stage of sleep our bodies need. This can leave us feeling tired the next day - no matter how long we stay in bed."

Researchers[22] reviewing all the scientific studies in this area concluded that alcohol intake (whatever the amount) increases your ability to get to sleep and gives you a better quality of sleep in the first half of the night, but it leads to more sleep disruption in the second half of the night.

You are unlikely to feel and function better the next day after drinking alcohol, so it's unwise to use sleep difficulties as an excuse to drink more.

CAFFEINE

Avoid drinking tea or coffee late at night. The Sleep Foundation[23] says:

"Caffeine enters the bloodstream through the stomach and small intestine and can have a stimulating effect as soon as 15 minutes after it is consumed. Once in the body, caffeine will persist for several hours: it takes about 6 hours for one half of the caffeine to be eliminated."

WHAT IF I CAN'T SLEEP?

If you can't sleep, get up and do something relaxing. Read, watch television or listen to quiet music. After a while, you should feel tired enough to go to bed again.

11

HOT FLUSHES/FLASHES/NIGHT SWEATS

*T*he UK charity breastcancer.org[1] says:
"Hot flashes have a lot to do with the changing levels of estrogen in your body, but other factors can cause your temperature control to go out of whack. Being aware of and addressing these factors can help you beat your hot flashes naturally. It may be tempting to look to medications right away - especially if hot flashes are severe - but try less drastic measures first. Severe symptoms should always be checked out to rule out a more serious cause, such as heart disease."

THE EFFECT OF LIFESTYLE

A study[2] of 17,473 postmenopausal US women, ages 50–79 women found that:

"... women who lost weight during participation in a dietary modification trial designed to reduce fat and increase fruit, vegetable, and fiber intake reported a reduction or elimination of VMS over one year. The dietary intervention appeared to ameliorate symptoms over and above the effect of weight change. These results support the use of weight loss and healthy dietary change as alternative approaches to hormone therapy for the relief of vasomotor symptoms."

A study in Chile[3] of 896 peri- and postmenopausal women found that various factors affected the hot flashes experienced by the participants. 58.5% were experiencing hot flashes. The main focus of the research was to look at the altitude the women lived at and how hot it was. But they also found that health and lifestyle affected the experience of hot flashes.

Women who were younger, in poor general health, had more depression and anxiety were more likely to experience hot flashes. Anxiety, temperature, lower life satisfaction, being older, taking regular strenuous exercise and a diet including regular hot spicy food affected hot flash frequency. Women who felt the hot flashes had a worse effect on their lives were on the whole anxious, having a lower life satisfaction generally, living at a lower altitude, taking less regular exercise and often feeling depressed.

Of course, it could be that women were anxious and depressed because of hot flashes, not the other way round. Unfortunately, the researchers did not address this problem.

BEING EMBARRASSED ABOUT HOT FLASHES

Psychologists and counsellors have found that those women who get most distressed about hot flushes often catastrophise the situation. This means they imagine the worse, making the situation seem increasingly frightening and out of control. Of course, when you think like this, your distress is likely to become worse. Women tend to assume everyone is just as aware of their hot flashes as they are themselves.

The UK Women's Health Concern website[4] from the charity the British Menopause Society offers a useful way to deal with the distress of hot flashes. (It also has a lot of other useful information.) The website suggests that you identify your negative thinking when you are experiencing a hot flash. You then think of ways to counteract this.

They suggest thinking: "This will pass soon". I found this simple thought really helpful when I was experiencing hot flashes.

If you are feeling that everyone is aware of your hot flushes, try thinking: "I notice my flushes more than other people, they may not notice". This is very likely to be true, as most people are far too much wrapped up in themselves to observe what other people are doing.

This idea that everyone is looking at you is called "the spotlight effect". You feel that everyone is focussing on you, examining you in minute detail. Feeling self-conscious can really undermine your self-confidence. It's very common to feel this way. But ask yourself this question: are people really this observant?

When you're feeling in the spotlight, name it. It's surprising how helpful that can be. Maybe you say/think something like this: "Oh here's me thinking again that I'm in the spotlight, when actually people aren't really thinking about me at all and they're not paying that much attention to what I'm saying or doing." This simple act of naming can be really helpful.

OWNING YOUR HOT FLASHES

You can decide, of course, to own your hot flashes and not try to hide them as if you are ashamed of them. What would this look like for you?

One of the ways I took the power away from hot flashes was by labelling them as "hotties". This name didn't suggest to me anything super-powerful. It suggested something slightly frivolous. Could you find a name for your hot flashes that takes some of their power away? I know some women like to call then "power surges".

THE ROLE OF STRESS

The other important aspect of hot flashes for me was when I realised that they occurred most and lasted longest when I was stressed. I came to see them as a message from my body (and mind) that it was under stress. Once the hot flash had passed, I would try to identify what the stress was so that I could remedy it. I'd ask myself various questions such as:

"Have I been eating badly?"

"Am I upset with someone and haven't resolved the upset?"

"Am I working too hard?"

If you take this approach, you start to see hot flashes as a helpful sign. A chance for you to change something to live more happily and healthily. If I'd taken HRT, I wouldn't have had these messages and would have lost my opportunity to make small corrections in my life. I learnt a lot of lessons then about what stresses me. Lessons I can still apply in my life even now the hot flashes have passed.

12

OSTEOPOROSIS

*U*sually, people start to lose bone density from around age 35. Oestrogen helps to make and rebuild bones. A woman's oestrogen levels drop after menopause, so bone loss speeds up. That's why osteoporosis is most common among older women, although men can get osteoporosis as well.

IS OSTEOPOROSIS NORMAL?

Is osteoporosis inevitable as you get older? People are more likely to suffer osteoporosis as they get older, but is it inevitable? Should we just accept that our fate as we age is crumbling bones and frailty? Should we resign ourselves to the possible fate of ending in an old people's home or nursing facility after a nasty fall?

The US National Osteoporosis Foundation[1] doesn't believe it is:

"Osteoporosis and the broken bones it can cause are not part of normal aging. There is a lot you can do to protect your bones throughout your life. You're never too young or too old to improve the health of your bones."

OTHER CAUSES OF OSTEOPORSIS

Menopausal hormone changes are not responsible for all cases of osteoporosis. If you smoke or are a heavy drinker, you are more likely to develop osteoporosis.

The North American Menopause Society[2] says:

"Heavy drinking can lead to osteoporosis that cannot be reversed. It's also a risk for fractures."

You may not have considered this. Even if you always drink expensive wine or spirits, you may still be a heavy drinker and be wilfully damaging your own health.

Some drugs[3] that can also lead to osteoporosis include glucocorticoids, proton pump inhibitors, selective serotonin receptor inhibitors, thiazolidinediones, anticonvulsants, medroxyprogesterone acetate, aromatase inhibitors, androgen deprivation therapy, heparin, calcineurin inhibitors, and some chemotherapies. Obviously, do not stop taking these drugs suddenly but consult your medical provider if you are concerned.

EXERCISE

If you have less robust bones, you are more likely to injure yourself if you fall. In the USA, falls are the leading cause of fatal and nonfatal injuries among older adults, causing hip fractures, head trauma, and death. According to Public Health England[4] around 20% of patients with hip fractures end up in long-term residential care within a year of the fracture.

A research review article by Doctors Barbara Sternfeld and Sheila Dugan in the academic journal Obstetrics And Gynecology Clinics Of North America[5] write:

"Regular physical activity is among the primary determinants of BMD [bone mineral density] and is a key contributor to overall musculoskeletal health, because of the responsiveness of bone to the mechanical forces that physical activities places on it. Both weight-bearing endurance activities, such as walking and running, and resistance exercises elicit this response."

The evidence for this is unequivocal. The UK NHS[6] says:

"It's medically proven that people who do regular physical activity have … up to a 68% lower risk of hip fracture [and] a 30% lower risk of falls (among older adults)"

Researchers from Leeds Metropolitan University[7] (UK) looked at research studies on the benefits of walking on post-menopausal bone loss. They concluded:

"… regular walking has no significant effect on preservation of BMD [bone mineral density] at the spine in postmenopausal women, whilst significant positive effects at femoral neck are evident. … Other forms of exercise that provide greater targeted skeletal loading may be required to preserve bone mineral density."

In other words, walking is not enough to preserve bone density after the menopausal transition is complete.

If you have osteoporosis and are nervous about exercising, check out the section in chapter XX on this specific point.

CALCIUM AND VITAMIN D

Calcium and vitamin D are also important for bone health. Many people advocate dairy as the best source of calcium. Some talk as though it's the only source of calcium. This, of course, isn't true. There are many people in the world who choose not to consume dairy products. This can be because their bodies do not produce the right enzymes to digest it. It can also be because they do not like the taste or associate the dairy industry with cruelty. Most of these people do not have poor bone health.

Dr Michael Greger reflects on dairy and calcium[8] in this way

"The #1 source of calcium in the American diet is dairy products. The #1 source of artery-clogging saturated fat is also dairy products; one of the top allergens in the U.S. food supply as well. So while cow's milk represents a substantial source of calcium, it comes with a lot of baggage. … The calcium in dark green leafy vegetables like kale, broccoli, and bok choy is absorbed about twice as well as the calcium in milk—and there's a bonus: fiber, folate, iron, antioxidants, and the bone-health superstar vitamin K. You won't find any of those in milk. What you do get as a bonus to the calcium in milk is saturated butter-fat, cholesterol, lactose, and antibiotics, pesticides, pus, and manure."

Vitamin D allows your body to absorb calcium and phosphate from your diet, which are essential for the development of healthy bones. Vitamin D is made by your skin on exposure to sunlight, but in some places, this is only significant for a few months of the year. You also need to be out in the sun and without sunscreen to get vitamin D this way.

You can get vitamin D from oily fish, red meat, eggs and fortified foods such as cereals. But the UK NHS[9] says:

" … since it's difficult for people to get enough vitamin D from food alone, everyone … should consider taking a daily supplement containing 10 micrograms of vitamin D during the autumn and winter."

It's interesting that the US National Osteoporosis Foundation[10] recommends eating fruit and vegetables for good bone health. People don't usually think about the importance of fruit and vegetables for bone health, but the research is there. Dr Michael Greger says[11]:

"Bone health isn't just about calcium; there are several key nutrients in vegetables, fruits, and beans associated with better bone mineral density. But, does that translate into lower hip fracture risk? The Singapore Chinese Health Study found that a diet rich in plant-based foods, namely vegetables, fruits, and beans, such as soy, may indeed reduce the risk of hip fracture."

Eat more fruit and vegetables! Does it sound familiar?

SLEEP AND BONE DENSITY

Dr Heather Ochs-Balcom and colleagues from the University at Buffalo found that chronic shortage of sleep has an effect on bone density. In their study 11,084 postmenopausal women, were assessed for bone mineral density (BMD) at four places on their bodies (whole body, total hip, neck, spine). Women who reported sleeping 5 hours or less per night had lower BMD for all four measures than women who reported sleeping 7 hours per night.

Dr Ochs-Balcom wrote[12]:

" ... women reporting 5 hours or less per night had 22% and 63% higher risks of experiencing low bone mass and osteoporosis of the hip, respectively. Similar results were seen with the spine. Our study suggests that sleep may negatively impact bone health, adding to the list of the negative health impacts of poor sleep. I hope that it can also serve as a reminder to strive for the recommended 7 or more hours of sleep per night for our physical and mental health."

UNDIAGNOSED COELIAC DISEASE

Research by George Mason University College of Health and Human Services found that adults who likely had undiagnosed celiac disease (UCD) had lower bone density than the adults without UCD, although they consumed more calcium and phosphorus. Lara Sattgast[13], one of the researchers, wrote:

"Our findings suggest that lower bone density among adults with UCD is not a result of their diets, and in fact, they took in more calories and nutrients than the control group. This may mean that these adults are not correctly absorbing nutrients."

If you have a suspicion that this could be you, ask your doctor about getting checked out.

ENVIRONMENTAL CHEMICALS

Another possibility is that chemicals are affecting your bones. Triclosan is an endocrine-disrupting chemical being widely used as an antibacterial in consumer goods and personal care products, including soaps, hand sanitizers, toothpaste, and mouthwash. You can be exposed directly by using these sorts of products or by drinking contaminated water.

Researchers published[14] their findings in the *Journal of Clinical Endocrinology & Metabolism*. They analysed data from 1,848 women in the US National Health and Nutrition Examination Survey to determine the link between Triclosan and bone health. They found women with higher levels of Triclosan in their urine were more likely to have bone issues. Yet another reason to swap out your personal care products for ones with fewer chemicals.

Looking after your bone health is part of a bigger picture of looking after your health and well-being so you can stay healthy and happy into old age.

URINARY INCONTINENCE

*U*rinary incontinence involves the loss of control of the bladder. For some women it's a small leakage of urine when they cough, sneeze, laugh or lift heavy weights. For other women it's a sudden urge to urinate that's so sudden and strong that they don't have time to get to the toilet.

Many women think that menopausal hormonal changes are likely to result in urinary incontinence, but the evidence doesn't support that.

ARE MENOPAUSAL CHANGES THE CAUSE?

A study published in the academic journal Menopause[1] doubted that menopausal changes were the cause of urinary incontinence, and that age was more important:

"After calendar age was controlled for, length of menopause showed no significant relationship with any symptom or sign of urinary incontinence.

"Conclusions: Hormone deficiency after menopause is unlikely to play a major role in urinary incontinence."

Being overweight or obese increases your chances of suffering from stress incontinence. Caffeine, alcohol and drinks with gas can also make the problem worse.

A Cochrane review[2] of the literature on oestrogen therapy for urinary incontinence in post-menopausal women concluded:

"Local oestrogen treatment may improve or cure incontinence. Data from two small trials, however, suggest that pelvic floor muscle training was more effective in the control of stress incontinence than local oestrogen."

PELVIC FLOOR EXERCISES

A review of the literature[3] on pelvic floor exercises supported their use for urinary incontinence:

"There is evidence for the widespread recommendation that pelvic floor muscle exercise helps women with all types of urinary incontinence. However, the treatment is most beneficial in women with stress urinary incontinence alone, and who participate in a supervised pelvic floor muscle training programme for at least three months."

Pelvic floor exercises strengthen the muscles around the bladder, bottom, and vagina (or penis for men). If you have trouble locating these muscles, try to stop the flow of urine when you are in the middle of peeing. Also imagine that you want to pass gas/wind and try to stop yourself. These are the muscles that are being targeted in pelvic floor exercises. Don't then practice your pelvic exercises while peeing. This exercise is just so you can locate them properly.

To strengthen your pelvic floor muscles, sit comfortably and squeeze the muscles 10 to 15 times. Do not hold your breath. Do not tighten your stomach, bottom or thigh muscles at the same time. Do this several times a day. Over time you will be able to hold each squeeze for a few seconds. You can also do more squeezes each time. You need to persevere to feel the benefits. There are lots of explanations and videos online, if you search for "pelvic floor exercises".

14

SEXUAL DESIRE

CW omen (and men) tend to find sexual desire decreases as they age. But some women report increased sexual desire, possibly because they no longer need contraception, and they may have more privacy if children have left home. It's important not to assume your sexual desire will lessen as you become menopausal. It's also important not to assume that a lower sexual desire will be a problem for you.

Hot flashes, night sweats and vaginal dryness can make intercourse more difficult. For some women the lack of desire is a problem in itself. For others it's a problem, because of the effect it has on their partner. The North American Menopause Society[1] report:

"... about 10% of US women are troubled by having low sexual desire. While a troubling lack of desire can affect women of any age, it has been reported in studies at a higher rate (12%) among midlife women (ages 45 to 64) than among women 65 or older (7%) or women younger than 45 (9%).

"Increasing evidence suggests that when women experience low desire, it's usually because of a number of factors rather than just a lack of sex drive. These factors may include issues or conflicts with their partner, medical problems, cultural issues, and others."

This quote talks about "a higher rate" among midlife women, but the absolute number is still not high. It also suggests that you should look at other factors and, once again, not just blame it all on your hormones.

VAGINAL CHANGES

*V*aginal dryness can occur at this time, but do not assume that this is the cause. Vaginal dryness can also be caused by perfumed soaps, feminine sprays, swimming pool chemicals, etc. Lack of arousal during sex can lead to vaginal dryness too. It's important also to exclude an underlying condition, such as diabetes or Sjögren's syndrome.

The Mayo Clinic[1] recommends various creams, lubricants, moisturisers and suppositories for this condition. The website also says:

"Regular sexual activity or vaginal stimulation - with or without a partner - also helps maintain healthy vaginal tissues in women after menopause."

HIGH BLOOD PRESSURE & CHOLESTEROL

*T*he charity bloodpressureuk.org[1] have a section of their website devoted to high blood pressure, menopausal symptoms and HRT. This is well worth reading.

Oestrogen has many protective effects. It helps to relax and dilate blood vessels, so blood can flow more easily. It decreases LDL cholesterol (the "bad" kind) and increases HDL cholesterol (the "good" kind). It also counteracts particles in the blood that can damage the arteries. As oestrogen levels drop, these beneficial effects lessen too.

These effects of oestrogen mean women have a lower risk of heart disease before menopause than men, but it rises afterwards. Also, if you've put on weight and are not sleeping as well, your chances of high blood pressure are raised.

TYPE 2 DIABETES

*T*he incidence of diabetes does go up as women age. It's not totally clear if any of this is attributable to the hormonal changes of menopause. The North American Menopause Society[1] says:

"But it does look like hormones do have something to do with it. If you are a woman over age 50, you're especially vulnerable, and women pay a heavy price for the disease. They lose more years of life than men with diabetes do. In addition, the death rate for women with diabetes has risen dramatically since the 1970s, while it has not for men with the disease."

The society isn't totally certain about the role of hormonal changes, but they definitely do not accept that it's all down to what happens at menopause. The Society recognises that being overweight and genetic factors play well-documented and important roles in the development of diabetes. It's definitely not all down to hormonal changes.

18

BRAIN FOG & MEMORY PROBLEMS

A study in Frontiers in Endocrinology[1] looked at 3,218 men and postmenopausal women. The researchers found:

"Postmenopausal women were at an increased risk of objective and subjective memory impairment than men."

Caroline Gurvich, Associate professor and Clinical Neuropsychologist, and colleagues from Monash University (Australia) write in an article on The Conversation[2] website:

"In most cases, it appears cognitive changes – that is, problems with thinking, reasoning or remembering – during menopause are subtle and possibly temporary… [but] they can raise concerns about developing dementia."

They go on to say:

"… menopause-related depressive and anxiety symptoms, sleep disturbance and vasomotor symptoms may make cognitive symptoms worse."

They also say that exercise can improve cognition during your midlife. They finish their article by saying:

"Avoiding illicit drugs, prescription medication overuse, smoking and excessive alcohol may be protective. A diet that

includes plant-based unprocessed foods (such as a Mediterranean diet), close social bonds and engagement, and a higher
level of education have been broadly linked to better cognitive
functioning during later life."

Does this sound familiar?

The UK charity Breastcancer.org[3] says that the mechanism
for how oestrogen levels affect mental functioning is not yet
understood. But the charity cautions against assuming any
memory problems are down to menopausal changes. They
could have other causes, such as stress, poor sleep, medication
or medical conditions. The charity goes on to say:

"The bottom line: If you're having memory problems, talk to
your primary health care provider, who can help you begin to
untangle possible causes.

19

DEPRESSION

a study of 221 US women[1] found that:

"Women were two to four times more likely to experience a major depressive episode (MDE) when they were peri-menopausal or early post-menopausal."

This study was just looking at the prevalence of it, not what precipitated it.

A study published in the academic journal Menopause[2] looked at 302 women's experience of a depressed mood during the menopausal transition and early post-menopause. The study lasted around thirteen years. The researchers found that women tended to be more depressed in the late menopausal transition stage. They also found that:

"Hot flash activity, life stress, family history of depression, history of "postpartum blues," sexual abuse history, body mass index, and use of antidepressants were also individually related to depressed mood"

This rather complicated picture can be summarised as the menopausal change itself did not trigger depression, except making women more vulnerable in the late menopausal transition stage. Other factors include body mass index and negative life events when they were younger had a bigger effect.

The North American Menopause Society[3] says:

"Women at menopause are especially vulnerable to depression, and heavy drinking can just make that worse. Heavy drinking itself can lead to depression, and women who show signs of alcoholism are two to seven times more at risk of developing depression than men."

Researchers from the Boston University School of Medicine[4] write:

"The mechanisms underlying the antidepressant effects of exercise remain in debate; however, the efficacy of exercise in decreasing symptoms of depression has been well established. Data regarding the positive mood effects of exercise involvement, independent of fitness gains, suggest that the focus should be on frequency of exercise rather than duration or intensity until the behavior has been well established."

20

ANXIETY & PANIC ATTACKS

*T*he UK Women's Health Concern website[1] from the charity the British Menopause Society says:
"Anxiety and stress are common reactions to everyday life. The menopause is not necessarily a stressful time, but it occurs during midlife when you may be dealing with other life challenges, such as parents' ill-health or bereavement, adolescent children, children leaving home (or not leaving home), or work demands. Having hot flushes and night sweats can also be stressful, and being anxious and stressed can make hot flushes more difficult to deal with."

The fluctuation of oestrogen and progesterone can cause feelings of anxiety or depression. But frequent, troubling high anxiety or panic attacks are not a normal part of menopause. It's important that you do not automatically blame hormonal changes, but seek professional help, as some women can develop a panic disorder at this time.

21

HAPPINESS & PURPOSE

*M*any women report feeling lost and uncertain and very tired as their hormones change. For some women children are leaving home. Maybe you look at your career and realise that you have got as far up the seniority ladder as you are going to get. These situations can make you sad, and it's easy to say that menopause is causing them.

You may need to work harder at being happy and positive during this time. Here are some suggestions for how to do that.

THE IMPORTANCE OF CURIOSITY

I love this quote from Robin Sharma

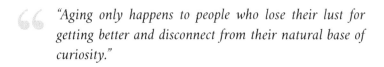

> *"Aging only happens to people who lose their lust for getting better and disconnect from their natural base of curiosity."*

Maybe he's exaggerating. Ageing does happen regardless of our mindset, but the speed and depressing nature of it can be restrained by a curious mindset.

I really think that curiosity is one of the most under-estimated beneficial mindsets. It seems to be even more important as we get older.

When you are curious, you find life more stimulating and enjoyable. When you are curious, you connect with other people better. When you are curious, life becomes more interesting and less boring.

You must know older people who are boring. They talk about a limited number of topics, maybe their ailments and their grandchildren. They aren't curious about the world, except maybe to say that it used to be so much better. They aren't really interested in you and what you are doing. People like this often feel lonely and invisible. They don't make the effort to reach out to other people, to be curious about them.

Curiosity is particularly important in this age of polarised views and information bubbles. Do you have friends who are different ages to you? Do you know and interact well with people who have very different political views to you?

It can be difficult, but curiosity can help you. Seek out people whose lives are very different from yours. Be curious about why they think the way they do. Try to understand how they experience life and how they interpret the latest news. Don't start from the point of trying to change what they think. Start by trying to understand how they see the world and their place in it. This can be hugely stimulating. If done honestly, it will probably encourage you to examine some of your own cherished views and certainties. And you'll have more to talk about with friends and family too.

Being curious about the world is also great for your brain. If you want to learn something new, try enrolling for a Massive Open Online Course (MOOC). MOOCs are free online courses available for anyone to enrol. They are often taught by academics or experts, who just want to share their passion. You can do a course on the fundamentals of statistics or learn more about food and health. Maybe you already speak some Spanish, but you want to learn more.

The easiest way to find a course is to search online using the word MOOC followed by the subject, so for example you would search "MOOC nutrition" or MOOC Spanish".

Curiosity can also help us be less judgemental about ourselves. This is vitally important as we age! Mindfulness is rightly hugely popular as a way of managing ourselves better. It can help you sleep better, be more relaxed, be less fearful and more contented. Central to mindfulness is the idea of curiosity – being curious about your thoughts, rather than trying to quell them with criticism and determination.

Curiosity can also help us to question the prevalent idea that we are going to become more passive and weaker as we get older. If you're curious, you won't accept the view that as you get older you will inevitably get more frail, more dependent and less yourself.

I love going to the gym and weight training. I'm really curious about how strong I can get. How much weight I can lift? Medication is seen as a normal part of ageing. I'm in my seventies. I'm curious to see if I can live my life without needing long-term medication by looking after my health and well-being.

Curiosity is ultimately non-judgemental of ourselves and others. It can give us a more interesting life, stimulate the brain and reduce cognitive decline. It can make us a supportive friend. Through curiosity we can seek to bridge the gap between ourselves and those we disagree with. We need a lot more of that in this world of strife and conflict.

TAKING DELIGHT IN SMALL THINGS

One of the big secrets of happiness is to take pleasure in small things. Many people belittle themselves for getting immense satisfaction from small things. You hear people say things like:

"I know it's sad but I get such a lot of satisfaction from ..."

The usual implication is that it's not a good thing to get satisfaction from small things. It shows a slightly shameful side to your character. Maybe it means you're shallow and not ambitious. But think about this again. Isn't it better to have small things that can give you a sense of happiness and satisfaction, rather than insisting on the big things? Focussing on achieving happiness in small things doesn't mean you can't achieve the big and dramatic things too. Having small go-to things that can make you happy is one of the keys to a happier life.

You almost certainly have some small things that are guaranteed to make you happy. What they are may be unique to you, but here are some possibilities:

- A tidy desk drawer
- A row of newly cleaned makeup brushes
- The colour purple
- Smelling roses
- Seeing a small bird
- Chopping onions finely

You may have to work at this if it doesn't come naturally to you, but it's so worthwhile. Getting pleasure in small things can give you little pockets of joy throughout the day.

WORK YOUR SKELETAL MUSCLES TO INCREASE YOUR HAPPINESS

I've already talked about the benefits of exercise during the menopausal transition.

Research[1] has shown that physical activity may help to "turn on" genes within skeletal muscles. This can then influence the key metabolic pathways that ultimately promote mood-enhancing chemicals within the brain, which help you to feel happy. Keeping our skeletal muscles strong helps to boost levels of the feel-good chemical serotonin, for example.

The problem is that as we get older our skeletal muscles tend to deteriorate. We feel more fragile, and we do less. This deterioration of our muscles influences those metabolic pathways, meaning that fewer happiness chemicals are produced. Fewer happiness chemicals mean less happiness.

Other research has also shown how exercise can improve our mood and reduce anxiety and depression.

VOLUNTEER TO BE HAPPY

Older people who volunteer are happier and healthier, so they are less likely to be depressed. It seems obvious when you think about it – volunteering means you are meeting new people, possibly learning new skills and feeling valued and needed.

A 2014 research project[2] confirms all this. The researchers reviewed 73 studies published over the last 45 years involving adults aged 50-plus who were in formal volunteering roles.

The review found that volunteering is associated with reductions in symptoms of depression and better overall health. Volunteers were also living longer than those who didn't volunteer.

They found that you need to volunteer for 2-3 hours per week to feel the benefit. Volunteering for more hours didn't increase these benefits but may still be what you want to do.

If you've got a chronic health condition you may feel volunteering isn't for you, but the research found that people like you benefited the most from volunteering.

SPEND TIME IN NATURE

Making time to be in nature, whether it's a local park, a hike or time spent in some wilderness area can be hugely beneficial.

Just sitting in your garden, if you have one, has beneficial effects too. If all else fails, look at the sky. Researchers have found that patients in hospital recover quicker if they have a view of the sky from their beds. Don't wait to be ill, get looking at the sky now.

Living close to nature and spending time outside has significant and wide-ranging health benefits according to researchers from UEA's Norwich Medical School[3](UK). They gathered evidence from over 140 studies involving more than 290 million people to see whether nature really does provide a health boost.

Their report reveals that exposure to greenspace reduces the risk of type II diabetes, cardiovascular disease, premature death, stress, and high blood pressure.

A study by researchers from the Max Planck Institute for Human Development[4] (Germany) found that time spent in nature positively affects the brain.

The researchers regularly examined six healthy, middle-aged city dwellers for six months. In total, more than 280 scans were taken of their brains using magnetic resonance imaging (MRI). The focus of the study was on self-reported behaviour during the last 24 hours and in particular on the hours that participants spent outdoors prior to imaging. In addition, they were asked about their fluid intake, consumption of caffeinated beverages, the amount of time spent outside, and physical activity, in order to see if these factors altered the association between time spent outside and the brain. In order to be able to include seasonal differences, the duration of sunshine in the study period was also taken into account.

Simone Kühn, head of the Lise Meitner Group for Environmental Neuroscience at the Institute said:

"Our results show that our brain structure and mood improve when we spend time outdoors. This most likely also affects concentration, working memory, and the psyche as a whole …"

22

HERBAL & OTHER REMEDIES

*T*he National Center For Complementary & Integrative Health[1] (USA) says:

"Keep in mind that although many dietary supplements come from natural sources, "natural" does not always mean "safe." Also, a manufacturer's use of the term "standardized" (or "verified" or "certified") does not necessarily guarantee product quality or consistency."

Dawn Ireland[2], a UK herbalist says:

"Using herbal remedies for the menopause is a complicated subject. The take home message for people is that there is no single remedy suitable for all. Everyone is unique. If your symptoms are challenging, the best option is to see a herbalist for a tailor made blend specifically for you. The blend may need changing over time as the body changes. Sometimes symptoms assumed to be menopause may actually be other issues, and it's good to check with your medical practitioner if symptoms persist.

"Peri-menopause and anovulatory cycles often brings temporary oestrogen dominance. This is because no ovulation means no feedback trigger to switch off the oestrogen which is building up. This can lead to longer gaps between periods, flooding and mood changes. The phytoestrogens in herbs (and in foods) are similar in shape but weaker than our own oestrogen. They attach to the oestrogen receptors in the body. This then lowers the impact of oestrogen dominance. Later when our own oestrogen production is very low, the phytoestrogens can mildly raise levels giving the body a boost. Not everyone has this pattern, and sometimes progesterone promoting herbs are also useful. A herbalist will work out which is the right combination for you."

It's important to buy supplements from a reputable supplier and not exceed the stated dose. If you are planning to use herbal remedies for the long-term, do consult a properly qualified medical herbalist. They will be able to advise about any potential toxicity concerns and herb-drug interactions.

Much of the research on herbal supplements is of poor quality or inconclusive. This is partly because there is no competitive advantage for manufacturers to support extensive research on herbs. Another reason is that often the research has used one herbal remedy and given it to all the women being studied. As herbalist Dawn Ireland has said everyone is unique. Herbalists will often give their patients a blend of herbs, changing it as the patient's experience changes. This more nuanced approach is difficult to apply in a research setting.

Having said all that, what does the research say about herbal supplements for menopausal symptoms?

BLACK COHOSH /ACTAEA RACEMOSA OR CIMICIFUGA RACEMOSA

A study in the Journal Of Education And Health Promotion[3] looked at black cohosh and evening primrose oil for hot flashes. The researchers concluded that:

"Both herbs were effective in reduction of severity of hot flashes and improvement of the quality of life, but it seems that black cohosh is more effective than primrose oil because it was able to reduce the number of hot flashes too."

A study published in the academic journal Maturitas[4] reviewed existing clinical trials and concluded:

"Black Cohosh appears to be one of the most effective botanicals for relief of vasomotor symptoms [hot flashes, night sweats].

The Women's Health Concern[5], a UK charity says:

"This North American traditional herb can help hot flushes although not as well as HRT. Black cohosh does not help with anxiety or low mood, but black cohosh can interact with other medicines and there are unknown risks regarding safety."

But another study published in the Annals Of Internal Medicine[6] concluded:

"Black cohosh used in isolation, or as part of a multibotanical regimen, shows little potential as an important therapy for relief of vasomotor symptoms."

Cochrane[7] is a not-for-profit offering "high-quality information to make health decisions". It reviewed 16 studies (involving 2027 women) and found insufficient evidence to support the use of black cohosh for menopausal symptoms. They went on to say that many of the studies were of poor quality and further investigation was needed.

So, should you try black cohosh? The evidence is mixed about whether it will be beneficial for you. You may want to try it and see if it helps you. If you do, buy it from a reputable source and do not exceed the stated dose. If you are taking medication, it's wise to consult a medical herbalist before taking it.

CANNABIS / CBD OIL

Smoking cannabis (marijuana) can make you quickly feel more relaxed and contented, so would seem like a good option at this time. But the long-term documented effects of cannabis should give you pause for thought. Cannabis may raise your chances of developing clinical depression or worsen the symptoms of any mental disorders you already have.

In a review paper in the academic journal Cannabis And Cannabinoid Research[8], the researchers conclude:

"... although some users may find [smoking] cannabis to be beneficial for ameliorating signs and symptoms commonly associated with menopause ... (e.g., insomnia, irritability, join pain, depression), there are few data on the efficacy and safety of cannabis use in this context."

They go on to point out that some of the research subjects were women who already smoked cannabis and had a favourable view of it from earlier in their lives.

CBD oil is extracted from cannabis but does not lead to intoxication or getting high. The website Medical News Today[9] reviews the action of CBD oil and says:

"There are cannabinoid receptors throughout the female reproductive system, and menopause seems to disrupt the endocannabinoid system. For these reasons, it is possible that CBD oil could reduce some symptoms of menopause."

It has been found to be beneficial for some forms of epilepsy. In the UK it's also prescribed for some multiple sclerosis sufferers, and for vomiting caused by chemotherapy. The research for its effectiveness for menopausal symptoms just isn't there.

If you decide to try CBD oil, it's important to buy it from a reputable supplier, as there aren't legal standards for its production, and then use with caution.

DONG QUAI

Dong Quai's Latin name is Angelica sinensis.

PeaceHealth[10] is a US not-for-profit. On their website they say that Dong Quai is known as the "female ginseng" and is sometimes sold as an aid for menopausal problems. They go on to say that this use is not supported by the Traditional Chinese Medicine system (TCM), where it's used for menstrual problems, such as painful menstruation.

I have been unable to find any recent research (less than 10 years old) that supports the use of Dong Quai for menopausal problems.

EVENING PRIMROSE OIL / OENOTHERA BIENNIS OIL

Evening primrose oil (EPO) contains high levels of omega-6 essential fatty acids. The word "essential" in its name tells us that it's something the body needs but cannot make itself. This is normally taken as a supplement in capsule form.

A research study published in the journal Archives Of Gynecology And Obstetrics[11] conducted a clinical trial with 56 menopausal women aged 45-59 years old. The participants were randomly assigned to take two capsules per day of a placebo or two capsules of evening primrose (500 mg) for 6 weeks. At the end of the six weeks the researchers asked the women about three aspects of hot flashes: frequency, severity and duration.

Both groups saw an improvement in all three aspects of hot flashes: 39%, 42 %and 19 %, in evening primrose group compared with 32%, 32% and 18% in the placebo group. As a result of the answers the women gave, the researchers calculated their Hot Flash Related Daily Interference Scales (HFDIS) and found that the percentage of improvement in social activities, relations with others, and sexuality was significantly superior to the placebo group.

FENNEL SEEDS / FOENICULUM VULGARE

A study published in the journal of the North American Menopause Society[12] looked at the effect of fennel seeds on the level of one of the oestrogen hormones (estradiol), menopausal symptoms, and sexual desire. The participants were divided into two groups. One group was given capsules containing fennel seed powder. This amounted to 2 gr (0.07 ounces) of fennel seeds. The other group was given a placebo. The experiment lasted 8 weeks.

The researchers concluded:

"The results of the present study indicated that daily use of fennel seed significantly improved menopausal symptoms in postmenopausal women over 8 weeks, though its effect on estradiol levels and sexual desire was not significant."

This was a small study of 80 women but taking fennel seed powder may be worth a try.

GINSENG / PANAX GINSENG

Researchers published a study of 72 postmenopausal women in the academic journal Menopause[13]. Half the women were given red ginseng (3g per day) and the others received a placebo. The trial lasted for 12 weeks. The researchers concluded:

"RG [red ginseng] could be an attractive herbal dietary supplement for relieving menopausal symptoms and conferring favorable effects on markers of cardiovascular disease in postmenopausal women."

KAVA-KAVA

Kava-kava is a herbal remedy that's made from the roots of Piper methysticum, which is a plant found in the islands of the Pacific Ocean. It's traditionally used to treat anxiety.

A review[14] of the research on this remedy concluded that it could be an effective treatment for short-term anxiety, but not as a treatment for long-term anxiety, particularly as there are concerns about its effect on the liver if taken for longer than eight weeks.

There have been limited studies of its use for the anxiety many women experience around the transition. A small study[15] looked at using Kava-kava alongside hormone therapy and reported a "greater reduction" in anxiety than for women treated solely with hormone replacement therapy.

So, should you try it? If you experience short bursts of anxiety, it may well be worth trying. If your anxiety is more long-term it's best to consult a medical herbalist rather than self-medicating.

PREBIOTICS & PROBIOTICS

Prebiotics are fibre and natural sugars that are found in some foods. They encourage the good bacteria in the gut. Probiotics are the actual gut bacteria which can be taken as a supplement or via fermented food.

A wide-ranging review of the influence of the gut microbiome on obesity published in the journal Preventive Nutrition And Food Science[16] found:

"… the use of probiotics and prebiotics improves gut bacterial composition and has achieved promising outcomes for prevention and treatment of obesity."

I think that over the next ten years there will be more and

more exciting research on prebiotics and probiotics. I think prebiotics will turn out to be more important than probiotics. Prebiotics provide the food that your existing gut bacteria need. More food means more bacteria. Prebiotics can be taken as a supplement, such as inulin capsules, or by eating the right food. Foods that provide higher levels of prebiotics include apples, asparagus, barley, unripe bananas, berries, flax seed, garlic, green vegetables, legumes (beans and peas), onions, and so on. Does it sound familiar? These are foods we've been talking about earlier in this book.

We may not understand the role of prebiotic foods for specific menopausal symptoms, but we do know that these foods are helpful for weight loss.

RED CLOVER /TRIFOLIUM PRATENSE

A review of the literature by researchers from Northwestern University[17] (USA) concluded that there was limited evidence suggesting that red clover supplements might be helpful for the maintenance of bone health and reduction in artery stiffness. They also found that at the moment there is no evidence that red clover is beneficial for hot flashes and night sweats.

ST JOHN'S WORT / HYPERICUM PERFORATUM

The Women's Health Concern[18] website says:

"St John's Wort was shown to have benefit in relieving vaso-motor symptoms, particularly in women with a history of, or at high risk of breast cancer. However, like black cohosh, it does interact with other drugs which again makes it a drug we have concerns about, including its reliability regarding dose effectiveness and safety profiles. Women on tamoxifen must not take St John's Wort as it makes the tamoxifen ineffective."

It also interacts[19] with other drugs, including anticoagulants, Ciclosporin, digoxin, and protease inhibitors used for HIV, specifically decreasing blood concentrations of these drugs.

23

COMPLEMENTARY &
ALTERNATIVE THERAPIES

*C*omplementary and alternative medicine are used by many women to help with menopausal symptoms. Many women are convinced of the benefit of this sort of approach. Yet the scientific evidence is at best uncertain.

This may be because much of the research is of a low standard. A large part of the reason for this is that there aren't the financial or institutional resources to do large scale clinical studies. There is no money for corporations in funding research, as there is nothing they can patent and monetise. I worked as a complementary therapist (kinesiologist) for many years, and I used to say that I was too busy getting people well to do the research that proved it was effective!

In an article looking at complementary therapies two professors[1] from Victoria University (Australia) write:

"Complementary methods such as acupuncture, moxibustion (a traditional Chinese medicine treatment that involves burning a herb called Mugwort) and reflexology are popular methods used to treat symptoms of various diseases, including menopausal symptoms.

"... there are contradictory studies, which some indicate that such complementary methods alleviate menopausal symptoms to some extent, while other studies demonstrate no benefit."

A review article by three Baylor University (USA) researchers in the Journal Of Evidence-Based Integrative Medicine[2] concluded:

"Results indicate that mind and body practices may be of benefit in reducing stress and bothersomeness of some menopausal symptoms. In particular, hypnosis is a mind-body intervention that has consistently shown to have a clinically significant effect on reducing hot flashes. Evidence is mixed in regard to the efficacy of natural products and there are some safety concerns."

ACUPUNCTURE

Some women have found acupuncture helpful for menopausal symptoms, but the scientific evidence has not shown this.

A Cochrane review[3] of the scientific literature on acupuncture for menopausal hot flashes concluded:

"When acupuncture was compared with sham acupuncture, there was no evidence of any difference in their effect on hot flushes. When acupuncture was compared with no treatment, there appeared to be a benefit from acupuncture, but acupuncture appeared to be less effective than HT [hormone therapy]."

Once again, we cannot conclude that acupuncture is not beneficial, only that scientific studies have not shown that it's for menopausal symptoms.

BACH FLOWER REMEDIES

The remedies were developed by Dr Edward Bach, who lived in England from 1886-1936. He was trained as a doctor and worked as a pathologist and bacteriologist, but he felt that medicine was not getting to the root of the problem. He learnt about homeopathy, and developed various important homeopathic remedies, but he was still not satisfied, and this led him to develop the Bach flower remedies. Although Dr Bach lived in England, his remedies are available worldwide. The remedies are based on flowering plants and trees. They are designed to correct inappropriate psychological states. This doesn't mean that they're not suitable for physical problems, because a positive psychological state can offer protection against physical problems.

Bach found the remedies through intuition: sometimes he would hold a flower in his hand and experience in his body and mind what the remedy was capable of, and sometimes he experienced deep negative emotions and would go out into the countryside searching until he found the flower that would turn off these feelings. Bach also found that if he floated the flowers in a glass bowl containing spring water in the sunshine, this healing property of the flower passed into the water. For some plants that flowered early in the year, such as holly, Bach boiled the flowers and stems to overcome the problem of the lack of sunshine.

There are 38 different flower remedies, each with its own psychological profile. Larch is for someone who lacks self-confidence. Aspen is for being generally fearful about lots of things in life. Heather is for people who want to be the centre of attention all the time. The remedies are usually provided in a dropper bottle and four drops can be taken directly into the mouth or they can be added to a glass of water and gradually sipped.

This may all seem a bit far-fetched and unlikely, yet there is some evidence that they work. A lot of this is anecdotal from enthusiastic users of the remedies, but there is also some research evidence. In my book "190 Weight Loss Hacks: What The Evidence Says" Hack 29 (Help With Binge Eating) describes a study using Bach Flower Remedies that was conducted at the Clinical Research Unit of the Medical School of São Paulo State University, Brazil. The results were published in the Journal of Alternative and Complementary Medicine[4].

One group was given a particular combination of flower remedies and the others had drops with nothing in them. The study lasted four weeks and the researchers found "an improvement in indices related to anxiety, sleep patterns, and binge eating" in the study group. You can read more about this in my book "190 Weight Loss Hacks".

A case study using a blend of Bach Flower Remedies was reported in the journal Alternative Therapies In Health And Medicine[5]. The participant was a 53-year-old, single woman, at the postmenopausal stage, who had been diagnosed with insomnia according to the criteria of the American Academy of Sleep Medicine. She was given a combination of flower remedies for four months. They used agrimony, gentian, olive, cherry plum, larch, walnut and white chestnut. The results were positive. She felt she was sleeping better, and objective sleep measures also showed that she was. Her menopausal symptoms and anxiety were also less.

So, which of the Bach Flower Remedies would be helpful for you? There are quite a few to choose from depending on your symptoms and experiences. There really isn't a menopause combination, because every woman's experience is different. Here are some of the ones most commonly used, but a quick search online will provide you with information on all of them:

Impatiens for tension and anxiety.

Larch for lack of self-confidence.

Crab Apple for inaccurate perceptions including of your own self-image. This remedy is useful if you are upset about the changes your body is going through or if you feel fat and ugly. It also may be useful if you are embarrassed or ashamed of your hot flashes.

Honeysuckle for a desire to return to a younger you, for wistfulness about your youth.

Pine for feelings of guilt and regret. You may regret missed opportunities or feel guilty about not spending more time with your family when they were young.

Hornbeam if you are tired and procrastinate a lot.

Olive is for complete exhaustion.

Walnut is for times of change and the need to adjust to new ways of being.

Cherry Plum if you are afraid that your mind is being over-strained and of your reason giving way.

White Chestnut for thoughts that go round and round preventing sleep and causing anxiety.

The remedies are normally taken in one of two ways:

- Putting two drops of the chosen remedy in a glass of water and sipping it frequently
- Putting two drops of one or several remedies in a bottle with water and/or brandy and taking 4 drops 4 times a day

Neither way is better. Do whichever is convenient for you.

There is one combination that Dr Bach found he used a lot, and he called this Rescue Remedy. This is a mixture of 5 of the 38 flower remedies (cherry plum, clematis, impatiens, rock rose and star of Bethlehem). It can be used for any emergency or stressful event. You can keep a bottle in a bag and take it as needed while you are out and about. If you don't have access to water, just put it straight in your mouth.

Since the work of Bach, other people have developed their own ranges of flower remedies. You can find more about those on the internet.

CHINESE MEDICINE

A Cochrane review[6] of Chinese herbal medicines for menopausal symptoms concluded that the studies did not produce good quality evidence on which to base conclusions about safety and effectiveness.

This, of course, does not mean that you won't find Chinese medicine helpful. It's just that there isn't enough scientific evidence that it's beneficial for menopausal symptoms.

COGNITIVE BEHAVIOURAL THERAPY/CBT

CBT is based on the idea that your thoughts, feelings, actions and even physical sensations are interconnected. Negative thoughts and feelings can lead to strange physical sensations and unhelpful actions, which increase the negative thoughts and feelings. This traps you in a vicious cycle.

CBT aims to help you manage problems that may seem overwhelming (or completely physical in nature) by breaking them down into smaller parts. By changing the way you think about your present situation you can change those reinforcing thoughts and actions and break out of the vicious cycle.

CBT, unlike some forms of therapy, focusses very much in the present and does not seek to find origins from your past including your childhood. This has led some to criticise it as not getting to the real core of the problem. But for many people a short course of CBT is financially viable and allows them to move forward practically in their current life situation.

CBT has been shown to be helpful for people who want to lose weight and for those with eating disorders. As with many approaches, it's best used as part of an overall plan to eat well and lose or maintain your weight.

The UK Women's Health Concern website[7] from the charity the British Menopause Society has a long detailed page on using

CBT for menopausal symptoms. This page is definitely worth a read, as it looks at how CBT can help various problems, such as anxiety, low mood, hot flashes and night sweats. The Society thinks that CBT can be very helpful for the menopausal transition. They see CBT as helping women think about the changes in a calmer way, meaning that they are then more likely to find positive steps to help with the symptoms they are experiencing. The Society says:

"Cognitive behaviour therapy is a brief, non-medical approach that can be helpful for a range of health problems, including anxiety and stress, depressed mood, hot flushes and night sweats, sleep problems and fatigue."

In a position paper[8] in 2015 the North American Menopause Society said:

"Cognitive-behavioral therapy and, to a lesser extent, clinical hypnosis have been shown to be effective in reducing VMS [menopause-associated vasomotor symptom – hot flashes and night sweats]."

ENERGY MEDICINE

Energy medicine modalities include homeopathy, kinesiology, light therapy and more. Many of these have not been tested according to standard scientific standards. Nevertheless, there are many women who are completely convinced that this type of therapy helps them feel better and have fewer distressing symptoms. These therapies are certainly worth exploring to see if they will help you.

HYPNOTHERAPY

In my book "190 Weight Loss Hacks: What The Evidence Says" I review the evidence on hypnotherapy and conclude that the evidence seems to suggest that hypnotherapy may be helpful for some people, but only alongside diet and lifestyle changes. The majority of hypnotherapists would not claim that you can lose weight just through hypnotherapy, but hypnotherapy can be helpful in making it easier to implement the changes you need to make in order to lose weight.

In a study[9] of 187 postmenopausal women reporting a minimum of seven hot flashes per day (or at least 50 hot flashes a week) participants who received five weekly sessions of clinical hypnosis reported a reduction in hot flashes.

Another study[10] reported that "hypnosis is a promising technique to improve sleep in menopausal women with sleep [disturbances] and hot flashes.

An article in the Journal Of Evidence-Based Integrative Medicine[11] says:

"… hypnosis is a mind-body intervention that has consistently shown to have a clinically significant effect on reducing hot flashes."

MINDFULNESS

Mindful eating is deservedly receiving a lot of attention. I've already talked in Chapter XX about how it can help you reduce your unhealthy eating without stressing you out. Can mindfulness help with specific menopausal problems?

In one study[12] 197 women were divided into two groups. One group took part in Mindfulness-based Stress Reduction program (MBSR), and the other group experienced a menopause education control program (MEC). The programs lasted 2 months.

The MBSR program used the normal mindfulness strategies and the MEC program gave health information, and exercise in a small support group.

The women completed questionnaires at the beginning of the study, immediately at the end of the programs after two months, then at five and eight months from the beginning of the study.

The researchers concluded:

"... menopausal symptoms in both MBSR and MEC significantly reduced over time of the study period of 8 months (6 months post intervention). MBSR show a greater reduction of psychological symptoms of depression and anxiety above active controls but similar reduction in somatic, urogenital and vasomotor symptoms."

So, both interventions worked, but the mindfulness training helped more with psychological symptoms than the menopause education control program did.

In an NCCIH-funded study[13], mindfulness meditation training reduced the "bothersomeness" of hot flashes in menopausal women and led to improvements in anxiety, perceived stress, self-reported sleep quality, and quality of life. However, the intensity of hot flashes did not change. Even though this study didn't show improvement in hot flashes, women who experienced them became less bothered by them.

All of this indicates mindfulness training should definitely be part of your toolkit for dealing with menopausal discomfort, as it has been shown to help with stress eating, sleep disturbances, anxiety and how you cope with hot flashes.

RELAXATION

A study by researchers at Southampton University[14] (UK) looked at women with primary breast cancer. 150 postmenopausal women diagnosed with primary breast cancer and who experienced hot flushes took part in the study.

One group of women received a single training session in relaxation based on deep breathing techniques, muscle relaxation and guided imagery. Over a month, they practiced relaxation for 20 minutes once a day at home using an audiotape.

They recorded the incidence and severity of hot flushes using a diary and validated measures of anxiety and quality of life. A second control group of women received advice on menopause management but no relaxation training.

The results show that, after one month, the incidence and severity of hot flashes in the group using relaxation techniques reduced significantly by 22% or seven flashes per week, compared to the control group which experienced no change. When examining the impact of flashes on the women's lives, the distress caused by the hot flashes was also seen to improve in the group using relaxation.

Cochrane[15] (UK not-for-profit) is less convinced:

"Evidence is insufficient to show the effectiveness of relaxation techniques as treatment for menopausal vasomotor symptoms, or to determine whether this treatment is more effective than no treatment, placebo, acupuncture, superficial needle insertion or paced respiration"

24

IS IT WORTH IT?

*Y*ou may be wondering if it's worth it. I'm suggesting you make lots of changes in your lifestyle. Some of them probably seem like hard work or even downright unpleasant.

You don't know how many years you've got left. You may feel that a short happy life is better than a killjoy life of food depravation and exercise boredom?

But the chances are that if you ignore the recommendations in this book, you won't have a short happy life. It's a very small percentage of people who are healthy and well and then one day drop dead. It's much more likely that you'll experience many years of ill health before you die. You may be in pain, breathless, afraid of falling, depressed. You may feel tired all the time and find everything a struggle. You may end up taking lots of medication and dealing with all the side-effects of that.

The actions in this book mean you are likely to have more healthy years in your life. These will be years in which you can still enjoy yourself and find a sense of purpose. If you have grandchildren, you'll still be able to play with them. If you want, you will still be able to play an active part in your community.

Of course, there are people who do all the right things, but still end up with chronic ill health. It's not a guarantee that you will have more healthy years. But doing these things gives you the best chance of being well into your seventies, eighties and even beyond.

I eat a largely healthy diet, avoiding sugary foods (most of the time) and drinking alcohol in moderation. I go to the gym regularly and use my bike to get around rather than the car. This is a healthy lifestyle. But if all it did was stop me putting weight on, I might not do it. Losing or gaining an extra few pounds isn't that important to me. But there are lots of other benefits of having a healthy lifestyle. It's these that make it totally worthwhile.

I wish I could bottle the feeling you get when you are feeding your body the right food and exercising regularly. If it was a medicine, you'd be clamouring for your doctor to prescribe it for you. Talking of medicine, there's a big satisfaction in not needing any!

When I went for an eye check-up recently, the optician said: "Any changes in medication?" The implication was clearly that I would be already taking medication. He looked surprised when I said: "No I'm not taking anything."

I had a check-up with a paramedic who was surprised that I wasn't taking any medication and that I had no chronic health problems. He told me I was doing "a good job". He recognised that my lifestyle plays a major part in this.

Exercising in the right way regularly gives you more energy. Exercise improves your mental state, reducing anxiety and depression. Regular exercise can reduce aches and pains, increase your confidence and reduce your chances of falling and breaking bones.

A healthy diet can reduce your chances of getting chronic diseases, such as type 2 diabetes. It can delay the onset of dementia. A healthy diet will stabilise your blood sugar levels, making you less vulnerable to mood swings and help you sleep better.

I've talked more about the benefits throughout the book. I want you to understand that you have a wonderful experience to look forward to that can be with you for the rest of your life. You can change your lifestyle without feeling deprived and miserable. A healthy lifestyle will probably mean you will feel happier for more of the time. Fighting menopause symptoms with drugs or simply accepting menopausal symptoms as inevitable won't give you that.

Drugs usually target one problem. Living well, sleeping well, exercising, losing weight targets your whole life. It's up to you. Even if you need to take drugs, living a healthy lifestyle will give you lots of benefits in terms of how you enjoy life.

And please do remember. You don't have to do it perfectly to feel the benefits. Make a start today and see how you get on. You may be surprised at how good you feel after making a few small changes.

THE EATING OUT ACTION PLAN

Do you struggle when you eat out? Do you end up eating more food than you want? Do you end up feeling weak-willed and fat? Then, is it difficult to get back on track? If this applies to you, my eating out action plan is what you need.

WORRY-FREE GUIDE: TO EATING OUT

I've brought together a 7-step action plan for when you eat out. Going to a restaurant or a party can be fun, it can also be very stressful, if you want to lose weight or keep off the weight you've already lost.

Each step is carefully explained. There's a bonus cheat sheet to take with you when you go out. You can either download and print it, or just have it accessible on your phone.

Download it here:
www.janethurnellread.com/freebie

LEARN MORE FROM JANE

www.janethurnellread.com- Jane's blog on health and well-being whatever your age.

@thrivingjane - Jane's Instagram account with pics of vegan food, inspiring tips and information, and videos of Jane in the gym.

Jane's YouTube channel - interesting interviews, short videos and more on health and wellbeing.

Check out more of Jane's books on Amazon

PLEASE REVIEW THIS BOOK

I hope you have enjoyed reading this book. If you have found it useful, please take the time to do a review on Amazon. It's so easy and quick:

1. Go to the Amazon page for this book
2. Scroll down to see the reviews.
3. Look for the button "Write a customer review" and click on that.

The more reviews there are for this book, the more likely Amazon are to show my book to prospective readers. You will be helping other people as well as helping me.

I read all my book reviews. I
would appreciate it if you
take the time to leave one for
this book. Thanks a lot.

ABOUT THE AUTHOR

I have been a university lecturer, a complementary therapist and an entrepreneur over the years. But throughout that time, I've had a love of books and writing. I enjoy sharing difficult information and ideas with other people in a way that doesn't dumb it down or disrespect people. People say that's one of my superpowers!

I'm now in my seventies – I'm fit, strong and healthy. That didn't happen by accident. In my twenties I drank heavily (a quarter of a bottle of whisky a day) and smoked around 40 cigarettes a day. My diet consisted of toast, chocolate and orange juice. I learnt bit by bit how to change that and become happier and healthier.

I believe that small changes can have big impact on our lives. I believe in offering practical information that you can apply in your life.

REFERENCES

1. INFORMATION IN YOUR HANDS & HOPE IN YOUR HEART

1. https://pubmed.ncbi.nlm.nih.gov/23847142/
2. https://www.maturitas.org/article/S0378-5122(15)30089-X/fulltext
3. https://thepsychologist.bps.org.uk/volume-24/edition-5/menopause
4. https://theconversation.com/post-menopause-hit-the-weights-not-the-treadmill-41809
5. https://www.pcrm.org/good-nutrition/nutrition-information/a-natural-approach-to-menopause
6. https://www.ncbi.nlm.nih.gov/pmc/articles/PMC6191885/

2. WEIGHT GAIN AT MENOPAUSE

1. https://www.monash.edu/news/articles/menopause-not-to-blame-for-weight-gain
2. https://www.healio.com/news/womens-health-ob-gyn/20220607/healthy-lifestyle-before-during-menopause-may-delay-severe-metabolic-conditions
3. https://www.sciencedirect.com/science/article/abs/pii/S0899900720302744?via%3Dihub
4. https://pubmed.ncbi.nlm.nih.gov/16491110/
5. https://theconversation.com/how-to-beat-weight-gain-at-menopause-123368
6. https://pubmed.ncbi.nlm.nih.gov/29216853/
7. https://www.sciencedaily.com/releases/2017/05/170531084443.htm
8. https://www.tandfonline.com/doi/full/10.3109/13697137.2012.707385
9. https://journals.lww.com/menopausejournal/Abstract/2017/09000/Does_obesity_increase_the_risk_of_hot_flashes.13.aspx

3. AM I TOO OLD TO CHANGE?

1. https://warwick.ac.uk/newsandevents/pressreleases/age_is_no
2. https://www.sciencedaily.com/releases/2019/08/190830082621.htm
3. https://www.betterhealth.vic.gov.au/health/healthyliving/Walking-the-benefits-for-older-people#bhc-content

4. WOULDN'T IT BE EASIER JUST TO TAKE HRT?

1. https://www.tandfonline.com/doi/full/10.3109/13697137.2012.707385
2. https://pubmed.ncbi.nlm.nih.gov/28898378/
3. https://www.nhs.uk/conditions/hormone-replacement-therapy-hrt/risks/
4. https://www.alzheimers.org.uk/about-dementia/risk-factors-and-prevention/hormones-and-dementia
5. https://ec.europa.eu/eurostat/statistics-explained/index.php?title=Healthy_life_years_statistics
6. https://theconversation.com/childhood-adolescence-pregnancy-menopause-75-how-your-diet-should-change-with-each-stage-of-life-132099

5. HOW TO AVOID MENOPAUSE WEIGHT GAIN

1. https://www.researchgate.net/publication/347315439_Morning_resolutions_evening_disillusions_Theories_of_willpower_affect_how_health_behaviours_change_across_the_day
2. https://www.sciencedaily.com/releases/2017/10/171002090509.htm

6. HOW CAN I AVOID REGAINING WEIGHT?

1. https://www.apa.org/science/about/psa/2018/05/calorie-deprivation
2. https://news.cuanschutz.edu/news-stories/cu-anschutz-study-reveals-exercise-is-more-critical-than-diet-to-maintain-weight-loss

7. CHANGING YOUR DIET

1. https://pubmed.ncbi.nlm.nih.gov/19661958/
2. https://pubmed.ncbi.nlm.nih.gov/30363011/
3. https://pubmed.ncbi.nlm.nih.gov/29704911/
4. https://careappointments.com/care-news/england/98121/new-survey-reveals-older-people-fear-dementia-more-than-cancer/
5. https://pubmed.ncbi.nlm.nih.gov/34274075/
6. https://bmjopen.bmj.com/content/9/12/e033038
7. https://journals.lww.com/menopausejournal/Abstract/2021/02000/Inverse_association_between_dietary_fiber_intake.8.aspx
8. https://nutrition.bmj.com/content/early/2019/08/27/bmjnph-2019-000034

9. https://europepmc.org/article/med/32979767
10. https://www.bbc.com/future/article/20190212-could-gut-bacteria-microbes-make-you-fat
11. https://www.theguardian.com/lifeandstyle/2018/mar/19/is-your-gut-keeping-you-awake-at-night
12. https://www.wcrf-uk.org/our-blog/could-you-eat-30-plant-based-foods-each-week/
13. https://www.health.harvard.edu/blog/theres-no-sugar-coating-it-all-calo-ries-are-not-created-equal-2016110410602
14. https://www.forbes.com/health/body/the-pulse-with-dr-melina/
15. https://www.ncbi.nlm.nih.gov/pmc/articles/PMC2765999/
16. https://www.bda.uk.com/resource/menopause-diet.html
17. https://journals.lww.com/menopausejournal/Fulltext/2021/10000/The_-Women_s_Study_for_the_Alleviation_of_Vasomotor.12.aspx
18. https://pubmed.ncbi.nlm.nih.gov/18328014/
19. https://www.ncbi.nlm.nih.gov/pmc/articles/PMC5808339/
20. https://www.nccih.nih.gov/health/providers/digest/menopausal-symp-toms-and-complementary-health-approaches-science
21. https://www.wcrf-uk.org/our-blog/could-soy-products-affect-my-risk-of-cancer/
22. https://journals.lww.com/menopausejournal/Abstract/2015/02000/Caf-feine_and_menopausal_symptoms__what_is_the.7.aspx
23. https://www.scirp.org/journal/PaperInformation.aspx?PaperID=2617
24. https://www.mayoclinic.org/healthy-lifestyle/nutrition-and-healthy-eating/in-depth/caffeine/art-20049372
25. https://www.caffeineinformer.com/
26. https://fdc.nal.usda.gov/fdc-app.html#/food-details/169593/nutrients
27. https://www.sciencedaily.com/releases/2020/05/200513121640.htm
28. https://www.unisa.edu.au/media-centre/Releases/2021/excess-coffee-a-bitter-brew-for-brain-health/
29. https://www.theguardian.com/lifeandstyle/2022/may/14/coffee-bad-red-wine-good-top-food-myths-busted
30. https://alcoholchange.org.uk/alcohol-facts/fact-sheets/alcohol-and-mental-health
31. https://www.mentalhealth.org.uk/your-mental-health/looking-after-your-mental-health/drink-sensibly
32. https://www.sciencedaily.com/releases/2021/07/210714110410.htm
33. https://www.hopkinsmedicine.org/health/wellness-and-prevention/alco-hol-and-heart-health-separating-fact-from-fiction
34. http://www.menopause.org/for-women/menopauseflashes/exercise-and-diet/drink-to-your-health-at-menopause-or-not
35. https://www.ncbi.nlm.nih.gov/pmc/articles/PMC1949018/
36. https://pubmed.ncbi.nlm.nih.gov/28074252/

8. BEHAVIOURAL CHANGE & MINDSET

1. https://www.sciencedaily.com/releases/2010/10/101018163110.htm
2. https://www.cdc.gov/healthyweight/losing_weight/getting_started.html
3. https://www.headspace.com/
4. https://www.amazon.com/dp/B09TQGVNWD
5. https://mbsrtraining.com/mindfulness-exercises-by-jon-kabat-zinn/mindfully-eating-a-raisin-script/
6. https://www.intuitiveeating.org/
7. https://www.sciencedaily.com/releases/2009/11/091104085230.htm

9. EXERCISE

1. https://www.garvan.org.au/news-events/news/why-women-should-eat-less-move-more-and-consider-wearing-transdermal-patches-during-menopause
2. https://michellesegar.com/why-you-should-stop-exercising-to-lose-weight/
3. https://www.psu.edu/news/research/story/menopausal-women-could-work-out-their-hot-flashes
4. https://www.ncbi.nlm.nih.gov/pmc/articles/PMC3270074/
5. https://www.sciencedaily.com/releases/2010/04/100405122311.htm
6. https://www.sciencedaily.com/releases/2017/02/170215084052.htm
7. https://www.sciencedaily.com/releases/2020/06/200608104727.htm
8. https://www.wcrf-uk.org/our-blog/exercise-always-a-pleasure-never-a-chore/
9. https://theconversation.com/standing-on-one-leg-is-a-sign-of-good-health-and-practising-is-good-for-you-too-168709
10. https://rightasrain.uwmedicine.org/body/exercise/exercise-snacking
11. https://www.lifehack.org/articles/lifestyle/you-hate-exercise-this-will-change-your-mind.html
12. https://www.nhs.uk/conditions/back-pain/treatment/
13. https://www.webmd.com/back-pain/ss/slideshow-exercises
14. https://www.bidmc.org/about-bidmc/wellness-insights/pain/2018/07/dont-back-down-from-back-pain
15. https://relaxtheback.com/blogs/news/exercise-with-back-pain
16. https://www.mayoclinic.org/symptoms/back-pain/basics/when-to-see-doctor/sym-20050878
17. https://www.prevention.com/fitness/fitness-tips/g20461557/relieve-back-pain-with-these-workout-tips/
18. https://hasfit.com/
19. https://www.cdc.gov/chronicdisease/resources/infographic/physical-activity.htm
20. https://www.sciencedaily.com/releases/2019/10/191016131226.htm

21. https://www.cancer.net/survivorship/healthy-living/exercise-during-cancer-treatment
22. https://www.cancer.org/treatment/survivorship-during-and-after-treatment/staying-active/physical-activity-and-the-cancer-patient.html
23. https://www.cancer.net/survivorship/healthy-living/exercise-during-cancer-treatment
24. https://blog.dana-farber.org/insight/2018/02/can-exercise-reduce-risk-cancer-recurrence/
25. https://www.sciencedaily.com/releases/2019/10/191016131226.htm
26. https://www.cancercouncil.com.au/cancer-information/living-well/exercise-cancer/
27. https://www.mayoclinic.org/diseases-conditions/cancer/in-depth/secret-weapon-during-cancer-treatment-exercise/art-20457584
28. https://bjsm.bmj.com/content/early/2022/04/24/bjsports-2021-104634
29. https://www.huffpost.com/entry/why-youre-actually-too-em_b_9233196
30. https://www.bda.uk.com/resource/menopause-diet.html
31. https://pubmed.ncbi.nlm.nih.gov/22992273/
32. https://chear.ucsd.edu/blog/top-11-benefits-of-strength-training
33. https://www.sydney.edu.au/news-opinion/news/2020/02/11/strength-training-can-help-protect-the-brain-from-degeneration.html
34. https://theconversation.com/post-menopause-hit-the-weights-not-the-treadmill-41809
35. https://hasfit.com/
36. https://www.health.harvard.edu/staying-healthy/the-health-benefits-of-tai-chi
37. https://pubmed.ncbi.nlm.nih.gov/27216996/
38. https://www.hindawi.com/journals/jar/2011/234696/
39. https://pubmed.ncbi.nlm.nih.gov/12966613/
40. https://www.escardio.org/The-ESC/Press-Office/Press-releases/tai-chi-shows-promise-for-relief-of-depression-and-anxiety-in-stroke-survivors
41. https://www.sciencedirect.com/science/article/abs/pii/S0965229916300395
42. https://www.ncbi.nlm.nih.gov/pmc/articles/PMC4110168/
43. https://newsinhealth.nih.gov/2019/11/yoga-health
44. https://www.sciencedaily.com/releases/2021/07/210728105640.htm
45. https://www.bbc.co.uk/news/uk-wales-47159652

10. INSOMNIA/SLEEP

1. https://www.sciencedaily.com/releases/2020/09/200915121310.htm
2. https://www.sciencedaily.com/releases/2020/11/201116075728.htm
3. https://theconversation.com/why-sleep-is-so-important-for-losing-weight-145058
4. https://newsinhealth.nih.gov/2013/04/benefits-slumber

REFERENCES

5. https://www.menopause.org/for-women/menopause-faqs-menopause-symptoms
6. https://pubmed.ncbi.nlm.nih.gov/31239118/
7. https://www.ncbi.nlm.nih.gov/pmc/articles/PMC4481144/
8. https://news.byu.edu/intellect/teens-not-getting-enough-sleep-may-consume-4-5-extra-pounds-of-sugar-during-a-school-year-says-byu-research
9. https://www.nhs.uk/live-well/sleep-and-tiredness/how-to-get-to-sleep/
10. https://www.health.harvard.edu/staying-healthy/blue-light-has-a-dark-side
11. https://www.nih.gov/news-events/nih-research-matters/artificial-light-during-sleep-linked-obesity
12. https://www.sciencedaily.com/releases/2019/07/190719173554.htm
13. https://pubmed.ncbi.nlm.nih.gov/29787483/
14. https://www.headspace.com/
15. http://doi.org/10.1089/ict.2022.29020.dli
16. https://www.rcpsych.ac.uk/mental-health/problems-disorders/sleeping-well
17. https://pubmed.ncbi.nlm.nih.gov/24720812/
18. https://www.rcpsych.ac.uk/mental-health/problems-disorders/sleeping-well
19. https://www.ncbi.nlm.nih.gov/pmc/articles/PMC4505755/
20. https://sleep.biomedcentral.com/articles/10.1186/s41606-020-00047-x
21. https://www.drinkaware.co.uk/facts/health-effects-of-alcohol/effects-on-the-body/alcohol-and-sleep
22. https://onlinelibrary.wiley.com/doi/abs/10.1111/acer.12006
23. https://www.sleepfoundation.org/nutrition/caffeine-and-sleep

11. HOT FLUSHES/FLASHES/NIGHT SWEATS

1. https://www.breastcancer.org/treatment-side-effects/menopause/treating-symptoms/hot-flashes/managing
2. https://www.ncbi.nlm.nih.gov/pmc/articles/PMC3428489/
3. https://pubmed.ncbi.nlm.nih.gov/22946508/
4. https://www.womens-health-concern.org/help-and-advice/fact-sheets/cognitive-behaviour-therapy-cbt-menopausal-symptoms/

12. OSTEOPOROSIS

1. https://www.nof.org/preventing-fractures/prevention/
2. http://www.menopause.org/for-women/menopauseflashes/exercise-and-diet/drink-to-your-health-at-menopause-or-not
3. https://www.ncbi.nlm.nih.gov/pmc/articles/PMC4206646/

4. https://www.gov.uk/government/publications/falls-applying-all-our-health/falls-applying-all-our-health
5. https://www.ncbi.nlm.nih.gov/pmc/articles/PMC3270074/
6. https://www.nhs.uk/live-well/exercise/exercise-health-benefits/
7. in this population.
   https://pubmed.ncbi.nlm.nih.gov/18602880/
8. https://nutritionfacts.org/video/plant-vs-cow-calcium-2/
9. https://www.nhs.uk/conditions/vitamins-and-minerals/vitamin-d/
10. https://nutritionfacts.org/video/prunes-for-osteoporosis/
11. https://nutritionfacts.org/video/prunes-for-osteoporosis/
12. https://www.sciencedaily.com/releases/2019/11/191106085440.htm
13. https://www.sciencedaily.com/releases/2019/10/191017121928.htm
14. https://www.sciencedaily.com/releases/2019/06/190625102414.htm

13. URINARY INCONTINENCE

1. https://pubmed.ncbi.nlm.nih.gov/24061048/
2. https://www.ncbi.nlm.nih.gov/pmc/articles/PMC7086391/
3. https://pubmed.ncbi.nlm.nih.gov/20828949/

14. SEXUAL DESIRE

1. https://www.menopause.org/for-women/sexual-health-menopause-online/sexual-problems-at-midlife/decreased-desire

15. VAGINAL CHANGES

1. https://www.mayoclinic.org/diseases-conditions/menopause/expert-answers/vaginal-dryness/faq-20115086

16. HIGH BLOOD PRESSURE & CHOLESTEROL

1. https://www.bloodpressureuk.org/news/news/blood-pressure-the-menopause-and-hrt-.html

17. TYPE 2 DIABETES

1. http://www.menopause.org/for-women/menopauseflashes/bone-health-and-heart-health/diabetes-hits-women-hard-at-menopause-beat-it-back

REFERENCES

18. BRAIN FOG & MEMORY PROBLEMS

1. https://europepmc.org/article/MED/35527998
2. https://theconversation.com/brain-fog-during-menopause-is-real-it-can-disrupt-womens-work-and-spark-dementia-fears-173150
3. https://www.breastcancer.org/treatment-side-effects/menopause/treating-symptoms/memory-problems

19. DEPRESSION

1. https://www.cambridge.org/core/journals/psychological-medicine/article/abs/major-depression-during-and-after-the-menopausal-transition-study-of-womens-health-across-the-nation-swan/C1492885FCBF9B68C0990E70845F4DF4
2. https://pubmed.ncbi.nlm.nih.gov/18176355/
3. http://www.menopause.org/for-women/menopauseflashes/exercise-and-diet/drink-to-your-health-at-menopause-or-not
4. https://www.ncbi.nlm.nih.gov/pmc/articles/PMC474733/

20. ANXIETY & PANIC ATTACKS

1. https://www.womens-health-concern.org/help-and-advice/factsheets/cognitive-behaviour-therapy-cbt-menopausal-symptoms/

21. HAPPINESS & PURPOSE

1. https://www.sciencedaily.com/releases/2019/02/190207111309.htm
2. https://www.sciencedaily.com/releases/2014/08/140829135448.htm
3. https://www.sciencedaily.com/releases/2018/07/180706102842.htm
4. https://www.mpib-berlin.mpg.de/press-releases/taking-the-brain-out-for-a-walk

22. HERBAL & OTHER REMEDIES

1. https://www.nccih.nih.gov/health/menopausal-symptoms-in-depth
2. http://www.torbay-herbalist.co.uk/
3. https://www.ncbi.nlm.nih.gov/pmc/articles/PMC5868221/
4. https://www.ncbi.nlm.nih.gov/pmc/articles/PMC1780040/
5. https://www.womens-health-concern.org/help-and-advice/factsheets/complementaryalternative-therapies-menopausal-women/
6. https://pubmed.ncbi.nlm.nih.gov/17179056/

7. https://www.cochrane.org/CD007244/MENSTR_black-cohosh-cimi-cifuga-spp.-for-menopausal-symptoms
8. https://www.ncbi.nlm.nih.gov/pmc/articles/PMC8380785/
9. https://www.medicalnewstoday.com/articles/322078#specific-benefits
10. https://www.peacehealth.org/medical-topics/id/hn-2080003
11. https://pubmed.ncbi.nlm.nih.gov/23625331/
12. https://journals.lww.com/menopausejournal/Abstract/2020/11000/The_-effect_of_Fennel_seed_powder_on_estradiol.13.aspx
13. https://journals.lww.com/menopausejournal/Abstract/2012/04000/Effects_of_red_ginseng_supplementation_on.15.aspx
14. https://www.sciencedirect.com/science/article/abs/pii/S1744388118301981
15. https://pubmed.ncbi.nlm.nih.gov/11085051/
16. https://www.ncbi.nlm.nih.gov/pmc/articles/PMC7333005/
17. https://www.scholars.northwestern.edu/en/publications/clinical-studies-of-red-clover-trifolium-pratense-dietary-supplem
18. https://www.womens-health-concern.org/help-and-advice/fact-sheets/complementaryalternative-therapies-menopausal-women/
19. https://www.ncbi.nlm.nih.gov/pmc/articles/PMC1780040/

23. COMPLEMENTARY & ALTERNATIVE THERAPIES

1. https://theconversation.com/trick-or-treat-alternative-therapies-for-menopause-18007
2. https://pubmed.ncbi.nlm.nih.gov/30868921/
3. https://www.cochrane.org/CD007410/MENSTR_acupuncture-for-menopausal-hot-flushes
4. https://www.liebertpub.com/doi/full/10.1089/acm.2020.0305
5. https://pubmed.ncbi.nlm.nih.gov/28323628/
6. https://www.cochrane.org/CD009023/MENSTR_title-chinese-herbal-medicines-menopausal-symptoms
7. https://www.womens-health-concern.org/help-and-advice/fact-sheets/cognitive-behaviour-therapy-cbt-menopausal-symptoms/
8. https://pubmed.ncbi.nlm.nih.gov/26382310/
9. https://pubmed.ncbi.nlm.nih.gov/23435026/
10. https://www.ncbi.nlm.nih.gov/pmc/articles/PMC7097677/
11. https://www.ncbi.nlm.nih.gov/pmc/articles/PMC6419242/
12. https://www.ncbi.nlm.nih.gov/pmc/articles/PMC5919973/
13. https://www.nccih.nih.gov/health/menopausal-symptoms-in-depth
14. https://www.southampton.ac.uk/news/2008/05/relaxation-may-be-the-key-to-relieving-menopausal.page
15. https://www.cochranelibrary.-com/cdsr/doi/10.1002/14651858.CD008582.pub2/full

Printed in Great Britain
by Amazon

86413406R00098